Implementing and Evaluating Genomic Screening Programs in Health Care Systems

PROCEEDINGS OF A WORKSHOP

Siobhan Addie, Meredith Hackmann, Theresa Wizemann, and
Sarah Beachy, *Rapporteurs*

Roundtable on Genomics and Precision Health

Board on Health Sciences Policy

Health and Medicine Division

The National Academies of
SCIENCES · ENGINEERING · MEDICINE

THE NATIONAL ACADEMIES PRESS
Washington, DC
www.nap.edu

THE NATIONAL ACADEMIES PRESS   500 Fifth Street, NW   Washington, DC 20001

This project was supported by contracts between the National Academy of Sciences and 23andMe (unnumbered contract); Accenture (unnumbered contract); Air Force Medical Service (FA8052-17-P-0007); American Academy of Nursing (unnumbered contract); American College of Medical Genetics and Genomics (unnumbered contract); American Medical Association (unnumbered contract); American Society of Human Genetics (unnumbered contract); Association for Molecular Pathology (unnumbered contract); Biogen (unnumbered contract); Blue Cross and Blue Shield Association (unnumbered contract); College of American Pathologists (unnumbered contract); Color Genomics (unnumbered contract); Department of Veterans Affairs (Contract No. VA240-14-C-0037); Eisai Inc. (unnumbered contract); Eli Lilly and Company (unnumbered contract); Health Resources and Services Administration (HHSH250201500001I, Order No. HHSH250); Illumina, Inc. (unnumbered contract); Johnson & Johnson (unnumbered contract); Marc Grodman (unnumbered contract); Merck & Co., Inc. (Contract No. CMO-170216-001875); National Institutes of Health (Contract No. HHSN263201200074I; Task Order No. HHSN 26300093): National Cancer Institute; National Human Genome Research Institute; National Institute of Mental Health; National Institute of Nursing Research; National Institute on Aging; and Office of Disease Prevention; National Society of Genetic Counselors (unnumbered contract); and Northrop Grumman Health IT (unnumbered contract). Any opinions, findings, conclusions, or recommendations expressed in this publication do not necessarily reflect the views of any organization or agency that provided support for the project.

International Standard Book Number-13: 978-0-309-47341-5
International Standard Book Number-10: 0-309-47341-1
Digital Object Identifier: https://doi.org/10.17226/25048

Additional copies of this publication are available for sale from the National Academies Press, 500 Fifth Street, NW, Keck 360, Washington, DC 20001; (800) 624-6242 or (202) 334-3313; http://www.nap.edu.

Printed in the United States of America

Suggested citation: National Academies of Sciences, Engineering, and Medicine. 2018. *Implementing and evaluating genomic screening programs in health care systems: Proceedings of a workshop.* Washington, DC: The National Academies Press. doi: https://doi.org/10.17226/25048.

The National Academies of
SCIENCES · ENGINEERING · MEDICINE

The **National Academy of Sciences** was established in 1863 by an Act of Congress, signed by President Lincoln, as a private, nongovernmental institution to advise the nation on issues related to science and technology. Members are elected by their peers for outstanding contributions to research. Dr. Marcia McNutt is president.

The **National Academy of Engineering** was established in 1964 under the charter of the National Academy of Sciences to bring the practices of engineering to advising the nation. Members are elected by their peers for extraordinary contributions to engineering. Dr. C. D. Mote, Jr., is president.

The **National Academy of Medicine** (formerly the Institute of Medicine) was established in 1970 under the charter of the National Academy of Sciences to advise the nation on medical and health issues. Members are elected by their peers for distinguished contributions to medicine and health. Dr. Victor J. Dzau is president.

The three Academies work together as the **National Academies of Sciences, Engineering, and Medicine** to provide independent, objective analysis and advice to the nation and conduct other activities to solve complex problems and inform public policy decisions. The National Academies also encourage education and research, recognize outstanding contributions to knowledge, and increase public understanding in matters of science, engineering, and medicine.

Learn more about the National Academies of Sciences, Engineering, and Medicine at **www.nationalacademies.org**.

The National Academies of
SCIENCES · ENGINEERING · MEDICINE

Consensus Study Reports published by the National Academies of Sciences, Engineering, and Medicine document the evidence-based consensus on the study's statement of task by an authoring committee of experts. Reports typically include findings, conclusions, and recommendations based on information gathered by the committee and the committee's deliberations. Each report has been subjected to a rigorous and independent peer-review process and it represents the position of the National Academies on the statement of task.

Proceedings published by the National Academies of Sciences, Engineering, and Medicine chronicle the presentations and discussions at a workshop, symposium, or other event convened by the National Academies. The statements and opinions contained in proceedings are those of the participants and are not endorsed by other participants, the planning committee, or the National Academies.

For information about other products and activities of the National Academies, please visit www.nationalacademies.org/about/whatwedo.

PLANNING COMMITTEE ON IMPLEMENTING AND EVALUATING GENOMIC SCREENING PROGRAMS IN HEALTH CARE SYSTEMS[1]

W. GREGORY FEERO (*Co-Chair*), Representative of the *Journal of the American Medical Association*; Faculty, Maine Dartmouth Family Medicine Residency Program, Fairfield, ME

DAVID VEENSTRA (*Co-Chair*), Professor, Pharmaceutical Outcomes Research and Policy Program, Department of Pharmacy, University of Washington, Seattle

NAZNEEN AZIZ, Executive Director, Kaiser Permanente Research Bank, Kaiser Permanente, Oakland, CA

GAIL GELLER, Director of Education, Berman Institute of Bioethics, Johns Hopkins University, Baltimore, MD

JEFFREY HANKOFF, Medical Officer, Cigna Healthcare, Glendale, CA

GEORGE J. ISHAM, Senior Advisor, HealthPartners; Senior Fellow, HealthPartners Institute for Education and Research, HealthPartners, Minneapolis, MN

MUIN KHOURY, Director, National Office of Public Health Genomics, Centers for Disease Control and Prevention, Atlanta, GA

BRUCE KORF, Wayne H. and Sarah Crews Finley Chair in Medical Genetics; Director, Department of Genetics, Heflin Center for Genomic Sciences, University of Alabama, Birmingham

CHRISTINE LU, Associate Professor, Department of Population Medicine; Co-Director, Precision Medicine Translational Research Center (PROMoTeR), Harvard Pilgrim Health Care Institute, Harvard Medical School, Boston, MA

MARCELLA NUNEZ-SMITH, Associate Professor, General Internal Medicine; Director, Equity Research and Innovation Center; Director, Center for Research Engagement; Core Faculty, National Clinician Scholars Program; Deputy Director, Yale Center for Clinical Investigation, Yale School of Medicine, New Haven, CT

JAMES O'LEARY, Chief Innovation Officer, Genetic Alliance, Washington, DC

CATHY WICKLUND, Past President, National Society of Genetic Counselors; Director, Graduate Program in Genetic Counseling; Associate Professor, Department of Obstetrics and Gynecology, Northwestern University, Evanston, IL

---

[1]The National Academies of Sciences, Engineering, and Medicine's planning committees are solely responsible for organizing the workshop, identifying topics, and choosing speakers. The responsibility for the published Proceedings of a Workshop rests with the workshop rapporteurs and the institution.

Roundtable on Genomics and Precision Health Staff

SARAH H. BEACHY, Director
SIOBHAN ADDIE, Program Officer
MEREDITH HACKMANN, Research Associate
REBECCA RAY, Senior Program Assistant

Board on Health Sciences Policy Staff

ANDREW M. POPE, Director
STEPHANIE YOUNG, Program Coordinator (*from January 2018*)

ROUNDTABLE ON GENOMICS AND PRECISION HEALTH[1]

GEOFFREY GINSBURG (*Co-Chair*), Director, Center for Applied Genomics and Precision Medicine, Duke University, Durham, NC
SHARON TERRY (*Co-Chair*), President and Chief Executive Officer, Genetic Alliance, Washington, DC
NAOMI ARONSON, Executive Director, Technology Evaluation Center, Blue Cross and Blue Shield Association, Chicago, IL
NAZNEEN AZIZ, Executive Director, Kaiser Permanente Research Bank, Kaiser Permanente, Oakland, CA
KARINA BIENFAIT, Head, Global Genomics Policy, Process and Compliance, Merck and Co., Inc., Kenilworth, NJ (*from January, 2018*)
REBECCA BLANCHARD, Executive Director, Genetics and Pharmacogenomics, Head of Clinical Pharmacogenomics, Merck and Co., Inc., West Point, PA (*until January 2018*)
RUTH BRENNER, Chief of Air Force Medical Support Personalized Medicine, Air Force Medical Support Agency, Falls Church, VA
ANN CASHION, Scientific Director, National Institute of Nursing Research, National Institutes of Health, Bethesda, MD
ROBERT B. DARNELL, President and Scientific Director, New York Genome Center; Investigator, Howard Hughes Medical Institute, Heilbrunn Cancer Professor and Senior Physician, Head, Laboratory of Molecular Neuro-Oncology, The Rockefeller University, New York, NY
BARRY DICKINSON, Director, Science and Biotechnology, American Medical Association, Chicago, IL (*until February 2018*)
JOSEPH DONAHUE, Managing Director, Global Life Sciences Research and Development, Accenture, Berwyn, PA
MICHAEL J. DOUGHERTY, Director of Education, American Society of Human Genetics, Bethesda, MD (*until August 2017*)
W. GREGORY FEERO, Representative of the *Journal of the American Medical Association*; Faculty, Maine Dartmouth Family Medicine Residency Program, Fairfield, ME
ANDREW N. FREEDMAN, Branch Chief, Clinical and Translational Epidemiology Branch, Epidemiology and Genetics Research Program, Division of Cancer Control and Population Sciences, National Cancer Institute, Rockville, MD (*until February 2018*)
MARC GRODMAN, Assistant Professor of Clinical Medicine, Columbia University, New York, NY

---

[1]The National Academies of Sciences, Engineering, and Medicine's forums and roundtables do not issue, review, or approve individual documents. The responsibility for the published Proceedings of a Workshop rests with the workshop rapporteurs and the institution.

Reviewers

This Proceedings of a Workshop was reviewed in draft form by individuals chosen for their diverse perspectives and technical expertise. The purpose of this independent review is to provide candid and critical comments that will assist the National Academies of Sciences, Engineering, and Medicine in making each published proceedings as sound as possible and to ensure that it meets the institutional standards for quality, objectivity, evidence, and responsiveness to the charge. The review comments and draft manuscript remain confidential to protect the integrity of the process.

We thank the following individuals for their review of this proceedings:

GILLIAN HOOKER, Concert Genetics
GEORGE MENSAH, National Heart, Lung, and Blood Institute (National Institutes of Health)
DEAN REGIER, University of British Columbia
ROBERT WILDIN, University of Vermont Health Network

Although the reviewers listed above provided many constructive comments and suggestions, they were not asked to endorse the content of the proceedings nor did they see the final draft before its release. The review of this proceedings was overseen by **MELVIN WORTH.** He was responsible for making certain that an independent examination of this proceedings was carried out in accordance with standards of the National Academies and that all review comments were carefully considered. Responsibility for the final content rests entirely with the rapporteurs and the National Academies.

Acknowledgments

The support of the Roundtable on Genomics and Precision Health was crucial to the planning and conduct of the workshop on Implementing and Evaluating Genomic Screening Programs in Health Care Systems. Federal sponsors are the Air Force Medical Service; Department of Veterans Affairs; Health Resources and Services Administration; National Cancer Institute; National Human Genome Research Institute; National Institute of Mental Health; National Institute of Nursing Research; National Institute on Aging; and National Institutes of Health Office of Disease Prevention. Nonfederal sponsorship was provided by 23andMe; Accenture; American Academy of Nursing; American College of Medical Genetics and Genomics; American Medical Association; American Society of Human Genetics; Association for Molecular Pathology; Biogen; Blue Cross and Blue Shield Association; College of American Pathologists; Color Genomics; Eisai Inc.; Eli Lilly and Company; Illumina, Inc.; Johnson & Johnson; Marc Grodman; Merck & Co., Inc.; National Society of Genetic Counselors; and Northrop Grumman Health IT.

The Roundtable on Genomics and Precision Health wishes to express gratitude to the members of the planning committee for their work in developing an excellent workshop agenda and the expert speakers who explored how progress could be made in integrating genomics into large-scale health organizations. The project director would like to thank the project staff, who worked diligently to develop both the workshop and the resulting proceedings.

Contents

xv

Boxes and Figures

BOXES

FIGURES

Acronyms and Abbreviations

ACA   Patient Protection and Affordable Care Act
ACO   accountable care organization
ACMG   American College of Medical Genetics and Genomics
AML   acute myeloid leukemia

CDC   Centers for Disease Control and Prevention
CFIR   Consolidated Framework for Implementation Research
CMS   Centers for Medicare & Medicaid Services
COAG   Clarification of Optimal Anticoagulation
CPIC   Clinical Pharmacogenetics Implementation Consortium
CRCP   colorectal cancer and polyposis
CSER   Clinical Sequencing Evidence-Generating Research

EGAPP   Evaluation of Genomics Applications in Practice and
             Prevention
EHR   electronic health record
eMERGE   Electronic Medical Records and Genomics Network

FH   familial hypercholesterolemia
FQHC   federally qualified health center

GINA   Genetic Information Nondiscrimination Act of 2008
GUARDD   Genetic Testing to Understand and Address Renal Disease
             Disparities

HBOC	hereditary breast and ovarian cancer
HIE	health information exchange
ICER	incremental cost-effectiveness ratio
IHC	immunohistochemistry
IGNITE	Implementing Genomics in Practice
LDL	low-density lipoprotein
MSI	microsatellite instability
NHGRI	National Human Genome Research Institute
NIH	National Institutes of Health
OMOP	Observational Medical Outcomes Partnership
PACS	picture archiving and communication system
PCORI	Patient-Centered Outcomes Research Institute
PCORnet	National Patient-Centered Clinical Research Network
QALY	quality-adjusted life year
SNP	single nucleotide polymorphism
UAB	University of Alabama at Birmingham
U-PGx	Ubiquitous Pharmacogenomics
UVM	University of Vermont
VA	Department of Veterans Affairs
VHA	Veterans Health Administration

1

Introduction[1]

Genomic applications are being integrated into a broad range of clinical and research activities at health care systems across the United States. This trend can be attributed to a variety of factors, including the declining cost of genome sequencing and the potential for improving health outcomes and cutting the costs of care. The implementation and sustainability of such genomics-based programs are often dependent upon securing funding and finding a genomic medicine champion to get the program started. The goals of these genomics-based programs may be to identify individuals with clinically actionable variants as a way of preventing disease, providing diagnoses for patients with rare diseases, and advancing research on genetic contributions to health and disease. Of particular interest are *genomics-based screening programs*, which will, in this publication, be clinical screening programs that examine genes or variants in unselected populations in order to identify individuals who are at an increased risk for a particular health concern (e.g., diseases, adverse drug outcomes) and who might benefit from clinical interventions (see Box 1-1).

Although the adoption of genomics-based screening programs has increased in recent years, there is still much to be determined about the

---

[1]This workshop was organized by an independent planning committee whose role was limited to identification of topics and speakers. This Proceedings of a Workshop was prepared by the rapporteurs as a factual summary of the presentations and discussion that took place at the workshop. Statements, recommendations, and opinions expressed are those of individual presenters and participants, and are not endorsed or verified by the National Academies of Sciences, Engineering, and Medicine, and they should not be construed as reflecting any group consensus.

BOX 1-1
Definitions Used by the Workshop Planning
Committee in the Context of the Workshop

- **Genomics-based screening programs**—clinical screening programs that have the goal of examining genes or variants in unselected populations in order to identify individuals at risk for future disease or adverse drug outcomes for which there are clinical actions to mitigate risk.
- **Health care system**—an organization providing medical care to a select population.
- **Population**—individuals who belong to a health system that has implemented or will be implementing a genomics screening program.

---

potential health benefits and possible harms of these programs and their effectiveness, safety, and clinical utility (i.e., the ability of a genetic test to improve clinical outcomes and add value to patient-management decision making). Many current genomics-based screening programs examine germline variability in specific genes that have been evaluated and recommended by groups such as the American College of Medical Genetics and Genomics (ACMG),[2] the U.S. Preventive Services Task Force (USPSTF),[3] and the Evaluation of Genomics Applications in Practice and Prevention (EGAPP) initiative.[4] These include variants that are associated with adverse drug reactions, hereditary cancers, and rare diseases. However, some health care systems are screening for additional variants that lack strong evidence of clinical validity (i.e., the accuracy and reliability of a test in identifying or predicting the biological and medical significance of the test result) and clinical utility. Another concern related to the early implementation of genomic screening programs is that while meaningful data are being generated, those data frequently remain siloed at each individual organization or laboratory that is carrying out screening. There is an opportunity to develop incentives to share clinical and economic data from genomics-based

---

[2]To view the ACMG's recommendations for reporting of incidental findings in clinical exome and genome sequencing, see https://www.ncbi.nlm.nih.gov/clinvar/docs/acmg (accessed January 10, 2018).

[3]A list of current U.S. Preventive Task Force Services Grade A and B recommendations is available at https://www.uspreventiveservicestaskforce.org/Page/Name/uspstf-a-and-b-recommendations (accessed January 10, 2018).

[4]Summaries of the recommendations from the EGAPP initiative are available at https://www.cdc.gov/genomics/gtesting/egapp/recommend/index.htm (accessed January 10, 2018).

screening programs as a way to advance the field, support more consistent reimbursement policies for genomics-based services and downstream care, and encourage additional health care systems to begin implementing similar programs if the evidence demonstrates that genomics-based screening programs are valuable to patients, providers, and health care systems.

On November 1, 2017, the Roundtable on Genomics and Precision Health of the National Academies of Sciences, Engineering, and Medicine hosted a public workshop to explore the challenges and opportunities associated with integrating genomics-based screening programs into health care systems.[5] The workshop planning committee provided definitions to help lay the groundwork for the workshop (see Box 1-1). One goal of the workshop was to further develop the ideas presented at previous Roundtable workshops that covered the economics of genomic medicine,[6] genomics-enabled learning health care systems,[7] implementation science–based approaches to genomic medicine,[8] and data sharing.[9] This workshop was developed as a way to explore the challenges and opportunities associated with integrating genomics-based programs in health care systems in the areas of evidence collection, sustainability, data sharing, infrastructure, and equity of access. Box 1-2 lists the specific workshop objectives that were developed by the planning committee.

When the Roundtable was established in 2007, conversations about using genomics in health care settings were very speculative and far from

---

[5]The workshop agenda, speaker biographical sketches, statement of task, and list of registered attendees can be found in Appendixes A, B, C, and D, respectively.

[6]Resources from the Roundtable's 2012 workshop The Economics of Genomic Medicine are available at http://nationalacademies.org/hmd/Activities/Research/GenomicBased Research/2012-JUL-17.aspx (accessed January 8, 2018).

[7]A learning health care system, as defined by the Institute of Medicine in 2013, is a "system in which science, informatics, incentives, and culture are aligned for continuous improvement and innovation, with best practices seamlessly embedded in the care process, patients, and families active participants in all elements, and new knowledge captured as an integral by-product of the care experience" (IOM, 2013, p. ix). Resources from the Roundtable's 2014 workshop Genomics-Enabled Learning Health Care Systems: Gathering and Using Genomic Information to Improve Patient Care and Research are available at http://www.nationalacademies.org/hmd/Activities/Research/GenomicBasedResearch/2014-DEC-08.aspx (accessed January 8, 2018).

[8]Resources from the Roundtable's 2015 workshop Applying an Implementation Science Approach to Genomic Medicine are available at http://www.nationalacademies.org/hmd/Activities/Research/GenomicBasedResearch/2015-NOV-19.aspx (accessed January 8, 2018).

[9]Resources from the 2012 workshop Sharing Clinical Research Data are available at http://www.nationalacademies.org/hmd/Activities/Research/SharingClinicalResearchData.aspx (accessed January 24, 2018). This project was a coordinated effort of the Forum on Drug Discovery, Development, and Translation; the Forum on Neuroscience and Nervous System Disorders; the National Cancer Policy Forum; and the Roundtable on Genomics and Precision Health.

BOX 1-2
Objectives Developed by the Workshop Planning Committee

- Examine the types of evidence being collected as part of genomics-based programs at health care systems, and consider near-term opportunities for advancing knowledge about the clinical utility of genomic screening.
- Discuss financial considerations associated with genomics-based programs, including available models to quantify value and return on investment.
- Explore new ideas for sharing economic and clinical outcome data via collaborative networks, and consider the necessary infrastructure and resources.
- Consider policy issues associated with the implementation of genomics-based programs in health care systems including ensuring equitable access, increasing the diversity of the participants, and facilitating data security and privacy.

---

reality, said workshop co-chair W. Gregory Feero of the Maine Dartmouth Family Medicine Residency Program. Now, he said, multiple health care systems both nationally and internationally have made the commitment to generate large amounts of genomic information in the context of clinical care and are beginning to use that information for population health management. Although the origin of each program is unique, best practices are emerging that can help organizations in the early stages of launching genomics initiatives. Developing evidence of clinical validity and clinical utility remains a challenge that might be met by collaboration across large health care systems, Feero said. Workshop participants were asked to look to the future, and to think about how to leverage existing programs to develop more robust data on how genomics may or may not improve the health of populations.

OVERVIEW OF CROSS-CUTTING TOPICS HIGHLIGHTED DURING PRESENTATIONS AND DISCUSSIONS[10]

A number of topics were discussed during the various workshop sessions and discussions as participants considered the different aspects of integrating genomics-based programs into health care systems. The issues

---

[10]This is the rapporteurs' summary of the workshop's main topics and recurring themes, drawn from the presentations, panel sessions, open discussions, and summary remarks by the moderators. Items on this list should not be construed as reflecting any consensus of the workshop participants or any endorsement by the National Academies of Sciences, Engineering, and Medicine.

highlighted below were drawn from individual speakers' remarks and the open discussions and are described further in the succeeding chapters.

Data Needs and Data Sharing

Additional data on clinical utility and cost effectiveness would support the implementation and sustainability of genomics-based screening programs. However, it is unlikely that the data collected by individual organizations carrying out these types of programs would alone provide the statistical power necessary to draw meaningful conclusions. Furthermore, said Debra Leonard, the chair of pathology and laboratory medicine at the University of Vermont Medical Center, the field has not yet determined exactly what data and metrics should be collected and shared. Throughout the workshop, participants discussed the types of infrastructure needed for effective data sharing, including the usefulness of common data models and data standards. Many existing data networks do not contain structured data on whether a clinical genomic test took place and what the test results indicated. Many of the workshop participants also discussed incentives for collaboration and data sharing, including funding, statistical power, economies of scale, risk mitigation, and shared solutions.

Measuring the Value of Genomics-Based Screening Programs

The value of genomic testing from a traditional economic perspective was discussed at length during the workshop, and individual speakers emphasized the need to develop quantitative measures and data to demonstrate to health care system leadership and decision makers the clinical utility and return on investment of genomic screening. Dean Regier, an assistant professor at the University of British Columbia, stressed the importance of also considering personal utility in value assessments. Personal utility is the value that individuals receive from genomic information apart from their health outcomes ("the value of knowing"). Regier presented a survey at the workshop that indicated that patients place a high value on the return of actionable findings but that many also want to receive incidental findings (unintentional discoveries of potential medical significance), regardless of whether the identified condition is treatable (Regier et al., 2015).

Community Engagement, Diversity, and Equity

Understanding patient and public perspectives could strengthen the development of genomic screening programs and help determine the utility of these programs for the intended population. Sara Knight, a professor in the division of preventive medicine at the University of Alabama at Birmingham, said that policies developed with public participation are more likely to be perceived as legitimate and trusted and are more likely to be implemented. Throughout the workshop individual speakers emphasized that typically underrepresented populations should be meaningfully engaged in developing genomic programs (see Chapter 5). Diversity, including of race, ethnicity, education, socioeconomic status, and material hardship, should be considered when designing genomic programs in health care systems.

Implementation of Screening Programs

The important role of health care system leadership in driving genomic screening programs was emphasized by several workshop speakers, including Leonard. The long-term sustainability of genomics-based screening programs was identified as a challenge, and approaches to leveraging existing systems and resources were discussed. The size of the current genetic counseling workforce may not be large enough to meet the needs associated with a broad implementation of genomic screening programs in health care systems, and workshop participants discussed the perceived shortage of genetic counselors, which could be due in part to resource-intensive service delivery models. Potential solutions to this challenge include exploring new care delivery models, and training other health care system and community members to deliver screening results.

Returning Results to Screening Participants

Returning the results of screening programs to participants presents several practical and ethical challenges, including special issues associated with returning results for children. In one example discussed, return of results was found to be the key motivator for participation in genomic screening, even though the number of participants who would directly benefit was generally modest. Participants want to have actionable findings returned; however, as was discussed, there is no clear, agreed-upon definition of what is actionable. Concerns regarding false negative and false positive results (leading to, respectively, false reassurance and unnecessary treatment) were also discussed, as well as issues related to understanding prevalence and penetrance. Several speakers emphasized that individuals undergoing genomic screening need to understand that a negative result does not exclude the possibility that they have a pathogenic variant, even among the genes being analyzed. Across the discussions, panelists highlighted the need for transparency and clarity for participants when implementing genomic screening programs for research purposes, as opposed to using the programs for clinical testing.

ORGANIZATION OF THE WORKSHOP AND PROCEEDINGS

This Proceedings of a Workshop summarizes the presentations and discussion that took place at the workshop. The workshop began with a presentation from Michael Murray, the director of clinical genomics at Geisinger Health Systems, who shared his insights on how genomic programs have been implemented to advance population health management, using the Geisinger MyCode program as an example. This was followed by additional presentations from representatives from two health care systems, a state-based program, and a panel discussion about the evidence considerations for integrating genomics-based programs into health care systems (Chapter 2). The second panel session focused on the financial and sustainability aspects of genomics-based screening programs (Chapter 3). A third panel discussed approaches to optimizing data sharing among early implementers of genomics-based programs in order to work toward demonstrating clinical utility (Chapter 4). The fourth panel session addressed issues of equity and ensuring the participation of all segments of the population that are cared for in health care systems as well as issues of data security and participant privacy (Chapter 5). In the final session of the workshop, a model for accelerating evidence generation for genomic technologies was presented, and members of a panel shared their final insights on the policies and infrastructure needed to enable data sharing across institutions. The workshop co-chairs then summarized potential action steps drawn from the workshop discussions for supporting the implementation of genomics-based programs in health care systems (Chapter 6).

This workshop is critically important as the field moves forward toward a vision of having genomics as part of everyday health care, said Geoffrey Ginsburg, the director of the Duke Center for Applied Genomics & Precision Medicine and a co-chair of the Roundtable on Genomics and Precision Health. However, there are still barriers associated with implementing genomics programs into health care delivery systems, Ginsburg said, and additional evidence will be needed to convince physicians to adopt, payers to reimburse, and patients to accept this new paradigm of health care. He called upon workshop participants to identify the action items needed to develop a learning health care system focused on genomic medicine and evidence development.

2

Evidence Considerations for Integrating Genomics-Based Programs into Health Care Systems

Highlights of Key Points Made by Individual Speakers

- Genotype drives phenotype, and the genome contains fundamental medical information that is not being used in medical care. Capturing this information would facilitate the promise of genomic medicine—to improve patient outcomes, population health, and the cost effectiveness of care. (Leonard)
- Broader genomic screening in the context of the health care system could identify a subset of individuals who are at high risk for certain serious conditions and who might benefit from intensive screening and management. (Murray)
- It is beneficial to partner a research center with a health care delivery system to allow for small-scale implementation and the identification of the potential benefits and harms of a particular intervention before a decision is made to adopt the program across an entire population. (Goddard)
- Research informs the implementation of genomic programs within the delivery system by identifying the potential benefits of the intervention, potential harms of the intervention, and implementation choices for the delivery system. (Goddard)
- It is important to avoid false reassurance and ensure that individuals who undergo genomic screening understand that a negative result (i.e., screening that does not indicate a pathogenic variant in a particular gene) does not exclude the possibility

9

that they have a pathogenic variant or that they will develop a related condition in the future, even among the genes being analyzed. (Korf, Murray)

- Given competing demands on the time of primary care physicians and the tendency to defer complex patient management to specialists, new systems may be needed for patient management during the return of results that does not involve educating primary care physicians in genomics/genetics. (Goddard, Murray)
- A system for aggregating data is needed to help capture information from implemented genomic medicine programs (e.g., the total cost of care and outcomes) though there will be data privacy issues that must be addressed while this system is being developed. (Korf, Leonard)
- Many patients are willing to have their genetic data stored and shared for research purposes, but they may have concerns about the possible effects on their insurance coverage and thus will avoid sharing genetic information with their primary care physician. (Korf)

To open the workshop, keynote speaker Michael Murray, the director of clinical genomics at Geisinger Health System, described his organization's MyCode initiative as an example of a genomic screening program, and he shared some of the lessons learned. This was followed by the first panel session, which focused on evidence considerations for integrating genomics-based programs into health care systems. Panelists shared examples of the types of clinical data and other evidence that are currently being collected by genomics-based programs at health care systems, and they considered opportunities for advancing knowledge about clinical utility. Katrina Goddard, a senior investigator at the Kaiser Permanente Center for Health Research, described some of the challenges faced in integrating genomic programs into the care delivery system at Kaiser. Bruce Korf, the Wayne H. and Sara Crews Finley Chair in Medical Genetics, a professor in and the chair of the Department of Genetics, and the director of the Heflin Center for Genomic Sciences at the University of Alabama at Birmingham (UAB) School of Medicine, shared lessons learned in implementing the Alabama Genomic Health Initiative, which is offering genomic analysis to 10,000 individuals in Alabama, returning clinically actionable results and compiling a research database and biobank. Debra Leonard, the chair of pathology and laboratory medicine at the University of Vermont (UVM) Medical Center, discussed the Genomic Medicine Program at the UVM Health Network, which intends to provide genome sequencing for all 1 million people who use the network as a way to improve patient outcomes and make care more cost effective.

LESSONS FROM A GENOMIC SCREENING PROGRAM: THE GEISINGER MYCODE COMMUNITY HEALTH INITIATIVE

The Geisinger Health System serves the rural northeast and north central parts of Pennsylvania and has recently expanded into southern New Jersey. The Geisinger MyCode Community Heath Initiative[1] started in 2007 as a biobank initiative, Murray said. More than 170,000 Geisinger patients have signed up for MyCode, and more than 90,000 have undergone whole exome sequencing thus far (Carey et al., 2016). The only inclusion criteria for joining MyCode is that one must be a Geisinger patient, Murray said, and enrollees are not recruited for any health or disease parameters. Murray noted that the rural region of Pennsylvania that Geisinger serves is overwhelmingly European Americans (more than 90 percent Caucasian), which limits the ethnic diversity of the study population, though the rural location does allow Geisinger to address some aspects of socioeconomic diversity. The expansion to the Atlantic City area in New Jersey is expected to bring additional ethnic and racial diversity to the study, he said.

In 2014 Geisinger entered a collaboration with Regeneron Pharmaceuticals to launch the DiscovEHR study,[2] which combines longitudinal electronic health records (EHRs) with DNA sequencing information to map genetic variation. The primary objective of the collaboration is discovery research, Murray said, and he referred workshop participants to a recent publication on gene variants and the risk of coronary artery disease as an example (Dewey et al., 2016). An important secondary objective of DiscovEHR for Geisinger is the clinical return of results to patients and their providers. The collaboration with Regeneron has enabled the whole exome sequencing and identification of secondary findings that the entire project builds on, Murray said. Support for the clinical confirmation and the return of results comes from multiple sources, including Geisinger internal funding, donor and foundation funding, and other grants. The model is not yet generalizable and sustainable, but Geisinger is working to create the evidence that would bring support. While there is currently no insurance payment for this work, payers have been supportive of covering cascade testing (identifying and screening family members of those at risk for certain genetic conditions), Murray said, as genetic testing in those

---

[1]For more information on the MyCode Community Health Initiative, see https://www.geisinger.org/mycode (accessed January 16, 2018).

[2]For more information about the DiscovEHR study, see http://www.discovehrshare.com (accessed January 10, 2018).

individuals is no different than genetic testing of anyone else who might warrant it based on risk.

Geisinger Return of Results Program

Exome data from the DiscovEHR study are assessed with a goal to identify secondary results of interest and importance to patients and providers. When a returnable variant is identified in the research data, it is clinically confirmed and then entered into the patient's EHR. Then, there are three essential steps that happen once a result is entered into an EHR, Murray said. The first step is communication and counseling. The patient's health care provider is informed of the genetic testing result 5 days before the patient is, so the provider can be prepared to advise the patient as needed. The patient is then directly notified and invited to participate further and meet with genetic counselors. A small number of patients have declined to continue participation when informed of their result, Murray said. The next step is for the patient to undergo condition-specific evaluation and management. The third step involves cascade testing of at-risk relatives, which Murray said multiplies the beneficial effect of the program since first degree relatives are at a 50 percent risk of having the same variant. The consent rate for MyCode with return of clinical results is 85 to 90 percent, and this high rate has been attributed to longstanding relationships with patients and trust of the system. It is made clear in the consent process that it is not possible to predict the impact of any results on such things as a patient's disability and life insurance. To illustrate the process, Murray shared the case of a Geisinger patient and her family, which was recently featured in *Science* (see Box 2-1 and Trivedi, 2017). At this time, results are only returned to adults, Murray said. Planning is under way to expand the program to include children soon.

Results are currently returned for 76 genes which are associated with 27 conditions. The initial phases of this project have focused on the Centers for Disease Control and Prevention (CDC) public health Tier 1 conditions of hereditary breast and ovarian cancer (HBOC), familial hypercholesterolemia (FH), and Lynch syndrome.[3] Within the cohort of about 50,000 individuals, 1 in 76 individuals (1.32 percent) was found to have a significant gene change that is associated with one of these three conditions, a frequency that Murray noted was higher than newborn screening, which produces a positive result to 1 in 800 individuals. Although the published literature suggests that the prevalence of these three Tier 1 conditions would be lower, Murray believes that this is a very conservative estimate of the

---

[3]For more information on the CDC Office of Public Health Genomics Tier Table Database, see https://phgkb.cdc.gov/PHGKB/topicStartPage.action (accessed January 16, 2018).

BOX 2-1
MyCode Genetic Screening and Cascade
Testing Case Example

A 57-year-old Geisinger patient (pink circle) participating in the MyCode initiative was informed that a *BRCA2* variant had been found incidentally within her genomic sequence. She reported that she had no personal or family history of breast or ovarian cancer; however, her

- maternal grandfather died of colon cancer diagnosed in his 70s (grey square on the right, directly above the pink circle);
- paternal grandfather died of lung cancer in his 70s (grey square to the left);
- father died of prostate cancer, which was diagnosed in his 70s (orange square); and
- brother died in his 30s after being diagnosed with pancreatic cancer, a *BRCA2* associated cancer (green square).

The Geisinger team advised her that it would be useful to reach out to her brother's children, Murray said. Screening revealed that two of her nieces have the same *BRCA2* variant (white circle with dot), and the late brother's DNA was therefore presumed to be *BRCA2* positive. The third niece tested negative for the variant, and her own daughter also tested negative.

The patient underwent the designated evaluation and was subsequently diagnosed with ductal carcinoma in situ, sometimes called stage zero breast cancer. Murray noted that this diagnosis is believed to have greater significance in the context of a *BRCA* variant than when diagnosed outside of that at-risk category. He added that the patient had never been offered testing, nor had anyone in the family, and at the time her brother had been diagnosed with pancreatic cancer in the 1990s, the association between pancreatic cancer and *BRCA* was weak and just being explored.

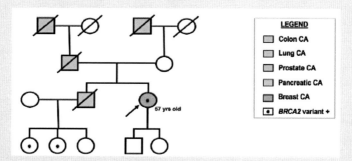

LEGEND
- Colon CA
- Lung CA
- Prostate CA
- Pancreatic CA
- Breast CA
- BRCA2 variant +

SOURCES: Michael Murray, National Academies of Sciences, Engineering, and Medicine workshop presentation, November 1, 2017. See also Trivedi, 2017.

number of people with genetic variants associated with risk for these conditions. Extrapolating to the total population of the state of Pennsylvania (12.8 million people), screening would be predicted to identify more than 150,000 individuals with positive genomic screens for these three conditions. The return of results process for the MyCode program is summarized monthly on the Geisinger website.[4]

The health care system is already set up to routinely screen for and prevent key elements of the CDC Tier 1 conditions (i.e., breast cancer, coronary artery disease, and colon cancer) without using genomic screening, Murray noted. Genomic screening could identify a subset of individuals who are at high risk for these conditions and who might benefit from intensive screening and management. Approximately 80 percent of those who were identified as having a *BRCA1* or *BRCA2* mutation as part of the MyCode screen had not been tested as part of their prior routine health care, Murray said. About half of those individuals met the criteria for genetic testing but had not been tested, and about half did not meet the criteria for testing. During the course of their routine care, about 20 percent had been offered and had received genetic testing for *BRCA1* and *BRCA2*. In other words, out of 50,000 individuals with an average of 14 years' worth of EHR data at Geisinger and hundreds of laboratory and other diagnostic tests on record, only one in five who screened positive for a *BRCA* variant had been previously identified through clinical testing.

Geisinger has been working to build the infrastructure to support the return of results, which includes, for example, a clinical genomics team, oversight committees, telemedicine, condition-specific multidisciplinary clinics, a family history tool, patient-centered genomics reports, condition-specific educational modules for clinicians, EHR tools, a provider liaison, and a cascade testing facilitator. Leadership within the Geisinger system, including the current chief executive officer, the former chief executive officer, and the chief scientific officer, is an important factor driving the genomic screening program, Murray said.

Lessons Learned from Genomic Screening at Geisinger

Based on the Geisinger MyCode experience, Murray said, there are several lessons learned that will help in planning for integrating genomic screening into health care delivery systems. First, genomic screening makes some invisible risks visible, as the family health history example of the 57-year-old woman who tested positive for a *BRCA2* variant shows. Second, traditional pretest genetic counseling for everyone undergoing screen-

---

[4]The return of results process for the MyCode program can be found at https://go.geisinger.org/results (accessed January 3, 2018).

ing will be difficult, given the nature of screening (i.e., the number of individuals expected to have a positive result) and the time needed for returning results to each participant. Third, unless or until it becomes a frequent event for a practitioner, primary care providers will, in most cases, defer patient management of screening results to specialists due to both practical time and expertise constraints. Finally, genomic screening will provide opportunities to correct clinical misattributions.

Genomic Screening Makes Invisible Risks Visible

Looking at FH as an example, Murray said that more than 40 percent of those in the 50,000-person MyCode cohort who screened positive for gene variants associated with FH had a low-density lipoprotein (LDL) cholesterol level below the typical cutoff of 190 that is used for diagnosis. This indicates that there is a large group of individuals who have the genetic change who would not be picked up within the health care system without this genetic finding, Murray said. Similar results have been published by others (Khera et al., 2016). Large studies have demonstrated that approximately 15 percent of people who present in emergency rooms or to health care providers with a myocardial infarction or acute coronary syndrome do not have identifiable risk factors for those conditions, and it seems clear that genetic risk such as FH will explain some of these cases, Murray said (Canto et al., 2011).

In response to a workshop participant's question about how receptive providers and patients are to receiving genetic screening information for FH, Murray said that there can be confusion about the relevance of the diagnosis of FH. People with very high cholesterol, for example, are already taking medication, and those with an LDL below the cutoff may not fully understand the disease and the need to have lower cholesterol goals than usual. In general, Murray said, the finding of the genetic variant provides an opportunity to intensify the management of these patients, and he pointed out that because Geisinger has a single EHR system, it is possible to track patients over time to determine if they are complying with recommendations for routine screening or other disease management.

Murray also described a second example in which a woman with no personal or family history received a positive BRCA result. Prophylactic oophorectomy in this patient revealed stage 1 fallopian tube cancer, which was removed. Treatment at stage 1 offers an excellent prognosis for this gene-associated cancer, which Murray said would not likely have been identified until the woman presented with symptoms at stage 3 or 4 if it had not been for the genomic testing.

Traditional Pretest Genetic Counseling Is Difficult

Before a genetic test is performed as part of clinical care, patients routinely meet with a genetic counselor and talk in great detail about what the test is, what it can show, and what the results do and do not mean. For MyCode enrollees, about 3 to 4 percent are expected to have a positive screening result returned to them, Murray said. For the other 96 or 97 percent who do not receive a positive result back, pretest counseling would not necessarily benefit them in the near term. As such, Geisinger is looking at other approaches to provide information to people without using 45 minutes of a counselor's time for each person enrolled in MyCode.

Primary Care Providers Are Likely to Defer Management

In the initial phase of the MyCode program, 270 notifications to providers were made. Of those, Murray said, 187 patient screening results went to internal primary care providers, 76 went to external primary care providers, and the remainder went to other providers. The 270 notifications went to 184 unique providers. This means that many primary care providers hear about the MyCode project for the first time when they receive these results. In almost every case, the providers ask if the Geisinger Genomic Medicine team can manage the patient, Murray said. There is educational support, and many providers have tried to learn more as a way to encourage their patients to follow up and to guide their patients to receive the right care. However, most primary care providers are not seeing a lot of MyCode patients, and they can refer them to a specialist as needed. "Where we really need to engage with [primary care providers] is in supporting the program and in taking the next step, such as preventing cancers or heart attacks," Murray said. He likened this scenario to how most providers in the United States do not see patients with positive skin tests for tuberculosis with any frequency and refer any such patients to an infectious disease or pulmonary specialist. For the foreseeable future, this is probably what will happen when providers see the occasional positive genetic screen, he said.

Correcting Misattribution Is Possible and It Matters

As an example of correcting misattribution, Murray described the first 14 MyCode patients who were identified as having hypertrophic cardiomyopathy gene variants. Seven had no diagnosis in their EHR and no history of having been evaluated for the condition. Seven had been evaluated, and two had been told prior to their genetic screening result that they had hypertensive heart disease causing their structural heart disease. The screening results showed that one of those people actually had non-obstructive cardiomyopathy resulting from a genetic change, not hypertensive heart disease. This finding has value not only to the patient, but also potentially to his family members. For the second person, both genetics and hypertension were found to be contributing. Misattribution is common within diagnostic clinical care, Murray said, and genetic screening identifies genetic changes, and provides an opportunity to rectify that misattribution.

One workshop participant asked how the leadership at Geisinger was thinking about penetrance of a disease in the long term. Murray said that they take a very stringent interpretation of genetic variants, which leads to high confidence that the pathogenic variants identified are a risk for driving clinical disease. Even so, some people with a pathogenic variant will not develop disease, and genetic counselors coach patients and providers on this. As data are collected over decades to come, the percentage of non-penetrance will become clearer, Murray said, and there are systems in place to reassess variants over time should the evidence level change. While some non-penetrance might be attributable to luck, he said, some will be because of biology, and there will be interesting research opportunities to determine if there are protective variants in families.

Exploring Challenges Moving Forward

In closing, Murray highlighted three challenges as the field of genomic screening advances:

- **Avoiding false reassurance.** The MyCode project has had to keep reinforcing the message that "no result means no result," Murray said. Not hearing back from the program does not mean that a patient is in the clear for a particular disease; it simply means that there was not a positive result signifying a significant risk among the genes that were screened. MyCode is a research program, and Geisinger strongly recommends that people who are at risk based on personal or family history have appropriate clinical testing done and be evaluated by the usual methods. Appropriately communicating the limitations of genetic screening will be important as the applications expand into public health or other similar settings, Murray said.
- **Understanding non-penetrance.** Currently, it is not possible to distinguish those individuals without disease who will eventually develop the disease from those without disease who will never develop it. Some individuals will have a risk variant and yet will go through life without ever developing the disease. It is important to make that message clear and to continue to work to better understand non-penetrance.

- **Making cascade testing work.** To be able to test first-degree family members where they live, Geisinger has worked with many clinical sites across the country, beyond the Geisinger system. The benefits of screening will be multiplied if systems for effective cascade testing can be implemented, but there is currently no roadmap for such testing.

INTEGRATING GENOMIC PROGRAMS INTO THE HEALTH CARE SYSTEM AT KAISER PERMANENTE NORTHWEST

Goddard described some of the challenges that Kaiser Permanente experienced with its genomic programs. Before offering several examples of these challenges, she highlighted three key areas of research that are being evaluated to inform the implementation of genomic programs within their delivery systems and listed examples of measurable outcomes of each program within the time frame of a typical research study. The first area is the potential benefits of the intervention, including patient management, information-seeking behavior of the patient, other changes to health behaviors, the potential for positive psychosocial impact, and change in health outcomes, which is typically not measurable within the time frame of a study. The second area being evaluated is the potential harms of the intervention, including negative psychosocial impact, misunderstanding, stigma or discrimination from receiving genomic results, health disparities, and costs associated with genomic tests. The third area is implementation choices for the delivery system, including impact on resources, workflow and logistical barriers, patient motivations and preferences, and the extent to which an intervention can be piloted before implementation.

Lynch Syndrome Screening

In 2011 Kaiser Permanente Northwest began a study on integrating universal Lynch syndrome screening into care for colorectal cancer patients.[5] Seventy-three patients were identified within the health system to evaluate whether Lynch syndrome screening resulted in a change in care management. The population prevalence of Lynch syndrome (1 in 440) suggests that around 1,100 people should have been identified in the region. The first barrier to be overcome, then, is the fact that people with these conditions are not being identified, Goddard said.

The study found that when patients do receive a result suggesting a diagnosis of Lynch syndrome, the patients and their providers would like a

---

[5]For more information on the study, see https://www.clinicaltrials.gov/ct2/show/study/NCT01582841?term=goddard&rank=5 (accessed January 10, 2018).

lot more support in care management. Nearly all of the 73 patients had a different primary care provider. Viewed another way, nearly all of the primary care providers likely have only one patient in their practice with this condition. Educating all of these primary care providers on the management needs for these patients is a large challenge, Goddard said, and she agreed with Murray about needing to rethink how patients with positive genetic screening results have their follow-up care managed.

Medical records were reviewed to determine what care was recommended for each of the 73 patients and how many actually received that care at the appropriate intervals (e.g., colonoscopy, endoscopy, genetic counseling, urinalysis, ultrasound, and other tests and procedures). Patient adherence (the extent to which patients received the recommended care at the appropriate intervals) was not 100 percent, and Goddard suggested that there is an opportunity to improve adherence to these recommended treatments.

Lynch syndrome screening among newly diagnosed colorectal cancer patients has now fully transitioned from a research program to a component of the care delivery system at Kaiser Permanente Northwest, Goddard said. The data from the research program provided the opportunity to show that genetic screening could be done systematically, she said. In addition, because the study randomized participants to either the usual care arm or the systematic screening approach, it was found that the majority of the people in the usual care arm (i.e., patient self-referral or provider referral to a medial geneticist) never went to geneticists and people with Lynch syndrome were not being identified.

The NextGen Study:
Examining Expanded Preconception Carrier Screening

One of the projects within the Clinical Sequencing Exploratory Research Consortium is the NextGen study[6] considering the impact of genome sequencing for expanded preconception carrier screening of women and their partners who are planning pregnancy in the near future. In particular, the study looked at whether there was a misunderstanding of "negative" preconception carrier screening results. In this context, Goddard explained, a negative result for a couple planning a pregnancy occurs when either the female partner was not found to be a carrier for any of the conditions, or the female partner is a carrier of at least one autosomal recessive health condition, but her partner is not a carrier for the same condition or was not tested.

---

[6]For more information on the NextGen study, see https://cser1.cser-consortium.org/projects/155 (accessed January 10, 2018).

This example helps to illustrate some of the potential harms that delivery systems are concerned about, Goddard said. One harm of particular concern was whether expanded carrier screening would lead to an increased use of health care services after genome sequencing (compared to those who did not receive genome sequencing or expanded carrier screening). The study assessed face-to-face, telephone, and e-mail encounters across primary care and mental health care. There were concerns about whether receiving carrier results might have some negative psychosocial consequences, Goddard said. The study found no difference between the two groups (genome sequencing versus usual care) in terms of overall use of health care services (Kraft et al., 2018). This could be reassuring to delivery systems to see that implementing an expanded carrier screening program would not lead to a significant uptake in unnecessary care services, she said. Another question that may arise is whether receiving carrier screening results will drive an increased use of mental health services, and in this particular study there was no evidence that people were seeking additional mental health services as a result of receiving their carrier results, said Goddard.

Another concern was whether women who had received negative carrier results would inappropriately decline recommended care during a subsequent pregnancy (e.g., ultrasound, amniocentesis, non-invasive prenatal testing, quad screen, other genetic testing). Again, Goddard reported, there was no difference between the two groups (genome sequencing versus usual care). Concerning refusals of pregnancy-related services, in one case the participant had declined a test because of a misunderstanding of her genetic test result, Goddard said. After a discussion with her provider, she decided to get the test that she had initially declined. This was only clear because the provider had documented it in the EHR, Goddard noted. In most cases it is challenging to understand the reasons for refusals as there is no documentation of them in the EHR.

Exploring Challenges and Opportunities Moving Forward

In closing, Goddard described several of the challenges she has encountered within her research studies and spoke about where more work may be needed to advance implementation. One of the challenges is that prospective studies have limited follow-up time during which to evaluate health outcomes, meaning that surrogates must be used. For patients, it is unclear what care can be attributed to the genetic test result as well as the reasons why care is refused. Another challenge is the lack of shared understanding of what is actionable genetic information, which Goddard said is one area where there is considerable opportunity to share information across programs and reach consensus. The Actionability Working Group of the Clinical Genome Resource, or ClinGen, a National Institutes of Health (NIH) resource, is focused on defining the clinical actionability of genetic variants. The working group is attempting to provide resources to the community to help build a consensus around what is actionable for each genetic disorder under consideration or, in other words, what are the well-established, clinically prescribed interventions that can prevent disease or delay the onset of the disease, lower clinical burden, or improve clinical outcomes.[7]

ALABAMA GENOMIC HEALTH INITIATIVE

The Alabama Genomic Health Initiative is a collaboration between UAB and the HudsonAlpha Institute for Biotechnology in Huntsville, Alabama.[8] The initiative had a $2 million allocation from the State of Alabama for 2017, with an additional $2 million for 2018, Korf said. The goal of the program is to offer genomic analysis to 10,000 individuals in Alabama in order to both return clinically actionable results and compile a research database and biobank.

Participants are being recruited into one of two cohorts. A population cohort of adults not selected for any particular phenotype is being given genotyping using the Illumina Global Screening Array, which Korf noted was chosen because of the low cost and adequate coverage of genes of interest. An affected cohort of individuals expressing phenotypes suggestive of a rare disease will receive whole-genome sequencing in an effort to achieve a diagnosis. Participants in the population cohort will be tested for variants of at least the 59 genes on the American College of Medical Genetics and Genomics list, although this may be expanded as the program develops. The detection rate of pathogenic variants is estimated to be about 50 percent, Korf said. Individuals who are positive for a pathogenic variant will receive free genetic counseling and will be connected to supportive longitudinal care based on their diagnosis. Participants in both of these cohorts will also have the opportunity to participate in the initiative's biobank effort, which will store DNA and other participant information for research use.

Initial funding was received in October 2016, and much of the period from October 2016 until May 2017 was spent getting institutional review board approval for the project and assembling working groups. Recruitment began on a pilot basis in May 2017 (with an initial 100 participants) and open enrollment began in July. More than 1,000 individuals were recruited from July to September 2017, and recruitment is continuing at the pace

---

[7]For more information on the ClinGen initiative, see https://www.clinicalgenome.org (accessed January 3, 2018).

[8]For more information on the Alabama Genomic Health Initiative, see https://www.uabmedicine.org/aghi (accessed January 3, 2018).

of about 100 people per week. Currently, participants have been enrolled from 45 of the 67 counties in Alabama. The age span of participants is 18 to 89 years, with enrollment numbers peaking in the 50 to 70 age group. Thus far, participants are about 73 percent female and 27 percent male, and 78 percent are white. The initial racial distribution during enrollment may have been a result of recruitment being done outside a major outpatient clinic at UAB, Korf said. Recruitment is now being expanded to other areas of the state, including Huntsville, Montgomery, Selma, and Tuscaloosa, to better mirror the state population.

During the consent process, individuals are asked whether they would like the results of their analysis to be shared with a primary care provider and whether they are willing to have their samples entered into the biobank. Nearly all participants (93 percent) consent to having their samples stored in a biobank; however, about half do not want their primary care provider to receive their results. Korf said that this might be the result of concerns about insurability. The program is now at the stage where it is beginning to return results. Every person that has an actionable or pathogenic finding will have genetic counseling provided, and counselors will be working to connect those people to providers who can help them to manage any risk that has been identified, Korf said.

For 2018, in addition to expanding recruitment to other regions of the state, the initiative is working to build trust in the community through the engagement of participants and providers and through public education about genomic medicine, Korf said. The initiative will also continue to develop the biobank and genomic database to support precision medicine research for years to come. Korf acknowledged the large number of people involved in the initiative, including an oversight committee, principal investigators, and working groups on bioethics, data and bioinformatics, education, genomics, and participant and provider engagement.

Lessons Learned by the Alabama Genomic Health Initiative

In the relatively short time that the project has been under way, Korf said that his team has learned valuable lessons, which he shared with the workshop participants, including comments about how his team is thinking about these issues as they move forward.

Adding Value for Participants

It is estimated that 1 to 3 percent of participants in the population cohort might receive an actionable or pathogenic result, Korf said. Because the global screening array only picks up about half of the potential pathogenic variants, fewer than 1 to 3 percent of participants would likely receive results, he said. Although the number of participants who will directly benefit is modest, the return of results and the potential impact of those results for an individual's family members does seem to be the key motivator for participation. The program has considered other approaches to add value for participants if needed, such as returning ancestry information, providing carrier status, or providing information about pharmacogenetic variants that might predict how a person responds to a medication. Korf noted that returning carrier status or pharmacogenetic information to the participants might require much greater genetic counseling capacity to meet the needs of those who receive this information. Furthermore, Korf said, it is likely that a participant will have long forgotten receiving a finding of a pharmacogenetic variant if the participant needs that particular drug in the future, and he raised a concern about potential liability for providers if that result is buried in a health record or lost due to the movement of patients among health care systems.

Concerns

There are various systems issues to be solved, including the need to increase the diversity of the population sampling, Korf reiterated. Another concern is that some people participate as a way of getting the genetic testing they need. The education and consent process is designed to make clear that people are participating in research, not clinical testing. Similar to points made by Murray and Goddard, Korf highlighted the education program's efforts to communicate that a negative result does not exclude the possibility that a participant has a pathogenic variant, even among the genes being analyzed (as the pickup rate is not 100 percent). If there is a clinical indication for counseling, it should happen in a clinical setting. The education program has recognized that this is an area that needs extra attention, he noted.

Impact

The Alabama Genomic Health Initiative is not just an opportunity to generate evidence, Korf concluded. It is also an opportunity to raise awareness and educate providers and citizens across the state to more readily embrace genomics as it matures in the future.

GENOMIC MEDICINE FOR THE UNIVERSITY OF VERMONT HEALTH NETWORK

The UVM Health Network serves about 1 million people in Vermont and northern New York. The network consists of six hospitals and the Medical Group, which is the network-wide physician organization, Leonard said. There is an affiliation agreement among the hospital network and UVM, the UVM College of Medicine, and the College of Nursing and Health Sciences. The network has also established two accountable care organizations (ACOs),[9] OneCare Vermont and AdirondacksACO, and OneCare Vermont has joined with two federally qualified health centers (FQHCs) to form the Vermont Care Organization. This is important, Leonard explained, because at the end of 2016 the state of Vermont signed an all-payer ACO model agreement[10] with the Centers for Medicare & Medicaid Services. The agreement calls for 70 percent of all eligible residents, including 90 percent of Vermont's Medicare beneficiaries, to be in an ACO or other value-based payment model by the end of 2022. Vermont is moving very rapidly from a fee-for-service model (where doing more results in more payments) to a global payment model focused on keeping people healthier, thereby reducing costs and accruing shared savings.

UVM Heath Network Genomic Medicine Program

Genotype drives phenotype, and a person's genome contains fundamental medical information that is not being used in medical care, Leonard said. The promise of genomic medicine, she continued, is to improve patient outcomes, improve population health, and improve the cost effectiveness of care, and this promise aligns with the current health care reform agenda in Vermont. Leadership at the health care system level is important for driving genomics programs forward, Leonard said, acknowledging the support of UVM Health Network chief executive officer, John Brumsted, in supporting genomic medicine for Vermont.

The vision of the Genomic Medicine Program in Vermont is to provide "genomes for all," that is, for all of the million or so people in Vermont and northern New York whom the UVM Health Network serves. The program has a clinical genomic medicine component, a genomic translational research component, and a genomic education component, all of them built around a number of central resources including a biobank, genome database, and health care database. When she was recruited as the chair of pathology and laboratory medicine, Leonard said, she received a half million dollars to start a genomic medicine program. An additional $2.7 million was allocated to build a laboratory for genomic medicine, with

---

[9]Accountable care organizations are groups of coordinated health providers that take responsibility for delivering high-quality care to patients. For more information, see https://www.cms.gov/Medicare/Medicare-Fee-for-Service-Payment/ACO (accessed January 16, 2018).

[10]For a further explanation of the Vermont all-payer ACO model, see https://innovation.cms.gov/initiatives/vermont-all-payer-aco-model (accessed January 16, 2018).

operational funding coming through the pathology and laboratory medicine budget from the UVM Medical Center. The genomic medicine team includes a director, four faculty members, a technical director, three technical staff, a genetic counselor and a pre-authorization specialist. Bioinformatics are handled through a partnership with PierianDx.

Clinical Genomic Medicine

The Genomic Medicine Program began genomic testing in 2016 with a cancer gene panel, the GenePanel Solid Tumor test, a screening panel for 29 actionable gene variants useful for diagnosis, prognosis, or treatment of solid tumors such as those in the breast, colon, and lung. The panel was initially ordered only by oncologists, Leonard said, but it is now being ordered by anatomic pathologists on all unresectable colon cancers, lung cancers, and melanomas (i.e., genomics has been incorporated into cancer care delivery). A rapid GenePanel for acute myeloid leukemia (AML) is currently being developed and validated. This needs to be a rapid test, Leonard said, because AML patients are very sick when they come to the hospital, and timely diagnosis is needed. A 100-gene panel for blood cancers (leukemia, lymphoma, multiple myeloma) is also being developed. In addition to cancer gene panels, a pharmacogenomics gene panel of 50 to 80 genes will be developed and will include clinical decision support built into the EHR based on the Clinical Pharmacogenomic Implementation Consortium guidelines. The next phase will move to exome or genome sequencing for inherited disorders, starting with patients with specific diseases or symptoms, such as cardiovascular disorders, neurologic/neuromuscular disorders, and unidentified inherited disorders in children. Additional patient cohorts will be added by disease type until, eventually, testing will be provided for everyone as long as the value can be demonstrated, Leonard said.

Genomics-Based Translational Research

Research on the clinical value of genomic testing is being done in collaboration with PierianDx, which is coordinating between Genospace, a cloud-based data storage and analysis platform, and Precision Health Economics, an economics research group looking at the value of precision health. This work is being funded by the UVM Health Network and the UVM Health Network Medical Group for an initial 2-year period, after which external funding will be needed, Leonard said. The available data that can be used to assess the value of genomic tests include genomic data, treatment and health outcomes data, cost data from claims and billing information, and patient demographics. For the GenePanel Solid Tumor test, for example, a recent (2013–2015) historical control group of solid-tumor patients will be compared to current solid-tumor cancer patients who have received genomic testing. Oncology care will proceed after the gene panel testing, and patients will be grouped according to the intervention received: (1) those that have received a targeted therapy, (2) those for whom no targeted therapy was indicated, and (3) those for whom targeted therapy was indicated but not given. Data from a 36-month period will be analyzed against the historical controls and among the three intervention groups for health outcomes (e.g., progression-free survival, overall survival, tumor response) and total cost of care.

Research is also under way on the implementation of genomic medicine and on functional genomics, Leonard said. The genomic medicine implementation research will identify issues for using genomics in clinical care, develop and implement strategies to address those issues, measure effectiveness and efficiency, and analyze and use the data and information. The functional genomic research will study biological impact variants of uncertain significance by building these variants into model systems to determine the functional effects and then provide that information to those involved in clinical care.

Genomic Education

Several ongoing genomic education activities are taking place at UVM, including an undergraduate honors college course called Controversies in Modern Genomics. For medical students, grant funding from the National Cancer Institute is being used to develop a national curriculum in genomics, and residents and fellows are learning about genomics as part of the molecular pathology rotation. To engage health care providers, 73 leaders across the UVM College of Medicine, Health Network, and Medical Center had their genomes sequenced through an Illumina Understand Your Genome program. The UVM Genomic Medicine Program is also hosting multidisciplinary conferences for health care providers to educate them about genomics through case study discussions that include researchers as well as specialists from applicable disciplines. To encourage patient, family, and public engagement and education, the Genomic Medicine Program is using a range of venues for outreach such as blogs, the press, community talks, and focus groups.

Potential Considerations Moving Forward

Evidence Generation and Data Sharing

The Genomic Medicine Program in Vermont is generating genomic data through genome sequencing, collecting other types of data (e.g., pathology, radiology, treatments, responses, costs), and using those data to assess whether a treatment for a patient was based on the genomic results received. While the information is not currently being shared with other organizations or health care systems, Leonard said, the genomic data could be submitted to ClinVar and ClinGen. A genomic cancer database is not yet available, nor is a place to share information related to the total cost of care. Leonard suggested that the *All of Us* Research Program at NIH could build a genomic medicine database to gather all of the data being generated by programs such as the UVM Genomic Medicine Program as a way to see the landscape of genomic medicine implementation across these systems.

Impact on Clinical Care

Prior to implementation of the genomic medicine program, other departments (e.g., pediatrics, obstetrics and gynecology, oncology, pathology, and laboratory medicine) were finding ways to address staffing and support for clinical genetics activities, Leonard said. They are currently developing a strategic and business planning process to better provide clinical genetics services across the UVM Health Network and to support the use of the genomic information that will be generated through the program, she added. The "genomes for all" approach to genomic testing will start with the testing of identified disease cohorts. In the all-payer model, test access is not based on an ability to pay. As such, the program does not foresee access issues based on ability to pay for the testing, and participation will be based more on patient choice. This begs the question of whether patient choice should be an option if, in a population health management model of care delivery, genomics does improve health outcomes and reduce costs, Leonard said.

Measuring Outcomes and Addressing Implementation Challenges

The important outcomes to measure depend on the purpose of the genome test, Leonard said. For cancer tumor response, progression-free survival and overall survival can be measured. For pharmacogenomics, adverse drug reactions, drug choice, and dosing adjustments can be assessed. For genetic disorders, diagnosis, secondary findings, and treatment options could be measured. The cost of care and of harms can be assessed for all. Tracking harms is not something that has been done thus far, Leonard said, but it is something that will be addressed as the program moves forward. She went on to say that if it is found that the program does not have sufficient value, it will be discontinued, although the hope is that the program will have value that can be demonstrated. Regarding challenges in implementation, Leonard said, one challenge that has been found is that oncologists are often not treating patients with the targeted therapy indicated by genomic testing.

DISCUSSION

Data Aggregation Across Programs

One workshop participant emphasized the magnitude of the amounts of data from genomic testing and the need to create a system to aggregate data from different programs, which is particularly important when dealing with rare diseases and even rarer genetic variants. Individual programs, even those that gather data from entire populations, will be limited in their ability to learn about rare conditions, Leonard said. That is, in part, why the focus of many genomic screening programs is currently on the more common, more prevalent variants and conditions. There are hurdles to overcome when aggregating data, including how to ensure data protection (i.e., patient privacy) and keeping the database updated, she said. Participants in the Alabama Genomic Health Initiative are given the opportunity to consent to having their information being used for future research, Korf said. This can include longitudinal data collection about outcomes in terms of both disease penetrance and screening and management activities undertaken as a result of the identification of the pathogenic variant. Korf also expressed support for the concept of a system for aggregating data. There is often a lack of evidence on the effectiveness of interventions that are undertaken following a genetic test result, Goddard said. In addition, when information about a specific population is not available, researchers often extrapolate from similar situations. Goddard noted the importance of defining what evidence needs to be captured when collecting and aggregating data.

Integrating Genomic Results into the EHR

A barrier to integrating genomics-based programs into health care is integrating genomic results into the EHR, a workshop participant said. In Geisinger's MyCode program, the genomic variant results of importance are entered into the problem list of the EHR, Murray said.[11] In this way, the result is always within the view of providers who might only open the chart casually or in urgent situations. For example, if a patient with a variant in a gene associated with long QT syndrome calls his or her physician on the weekend complaining of heart palpitations and instead reaches the provider

---

[11]The problem list in an EHR is the section where the most important health concerns for a patient are listed.

on call, that provider will see the genomic finding in the problem list and send the patient to the emergency department to be evaluated, rather than telling the patient to call back on Monday. The UVM Health Network is working with Epic to develop a standardized EHR for use across the health network, Leonard said. It is also providing input as part of Epic's molecular genomics workgroup. There is no single EHR in use across the state in Alabama, Korf said, and the Alabama Genomic Health Initiative has no control over entry of information into the EHR. Much of the communication is on paper, and the focus is on making sure anyone who has a positive result for a pathogenic variant is connected to a management plan.

Clinical Responsibility for Returning Reinterpreted Results

What is the responsibility downstream, one workshop participant asked, if there is a reinterpretation of variants or new evidence? For the Alabama Genomic Health program, Korf said, it was thought that attempting to keep participants informed on a regular basis was a daunting task. People frequently move, and there is often no way to re-contact them after their initial participation. The consent process is explicit in describing the screening as a one-point-in-time encounter, and it explains that, although knowledge is likely to change over time, the program cannot promise that it will be able to contact participants if something relevant to their profiles does change. There is an opportunity for participants to stay in touch with the program, he added, and if they want reinterpretation or would like to talk to someone about the significance of the results, that can be arranged, though the onus is on them as the participants. For the program at Geisinger, there are no systems or budget for re-contacting participants. Because all participants are in the Geisinger health care and EHR system, it could be possible to reach them in the future, but there is no promise made of a continuous review of results into the future. Systems are not yet in place for long-term re-contact, Goddard agreed, though it is also important to make sure that people understand that their results may be different if they are tested again in the future. Because the testing in Vermont is being done in a clinical setting, the plan is to build in reanalysis and send new results to health care providers, genetic counselors, and medical geneticists who would be responsible for reporting those results to participants, Leonard said.

Demonstrating Utility

A theme that arose multiple times during the discussion was the importance of institutional leadership support for genomics-based programs. There is an opportunity cost to investing in genomics (i.e., money that is invested in genomics could have been invested elsewhere), and all of the program leaders have a vested interest in demonstrating the utility of genomic testing, said a workshop participant who went on to ask how the programs plan to measure the long-term added value of benefits versus harms so that their institutional leadership will continue to support the programs. The Alabama Genomic Health Initiative is not designed to be a test of the value of genomic medicine, Korf said. Rather, it is a test of the particular approach that is being tried in a state which, historically, has not had many large community health programs. Program leaders have been cautious and measured in what has been promised. If realistic expectations are set, then a set of questions can be answered, he said. Kaiser collaborates with FQHCs, Goddard said, which have extremely limited resources and approach genomic testing in terms of the opportunity costs (i.e., what else their providers could be doing for their patients instead of genomic screening). Patients and providers in those systems have emphasized the importance of equity, noting that if genomic solutions are available in other health care settings, they would like to also see them implemented within their systems. Leonard explained that she was given a 10-year window in which to demonstrate utility because, during discussions of setting up the laboratory, she suggested to leadership that in 10 years the Genomic Medicine Program would be sequencing the genome of every patient who comes through the health network. Her leadership agreed and was willing to integrate genome sequencing into the clinical laboratory in the health network so that the process would be ready when the evidence was available.

Panelists were asked to think about how to combine their data with data from other institutions with genomics-based programs in order to provide the economic evidence needed for other health care systems to initiate their own genomic programs. Perhaps, a workshop participant said, an economic model could be developed of the outcomes that would be expected in Lynch syndrome or HBOC over time in the absence versus in the presence of the data already generated by genomics-based programs. The Alabama Genomic Health Initiative would welcome an opportunity to be networked into a larger community and share data, Korf said. The array that the initiative is currently using has a lower sensitivity but an affordable cost per patient, which could potentially translate to large-scale screening if the initiative can demonstrate cost effectiveness. Different systems are doing genomic testing in different ways, Leonard said, and while some are testing in a clinical setting where there are EHR outcomes and cost data, others are not. Any coalescing of data should be among systems that have EHR data and cost data (i.e., billing and claims data) so that both outcomes and financial impacts can be measured, Leonard said.

Genomic Testing as an Essential Health Benefit

Including genomic testing as an essential covered health benefit[12] would make it more widely available to more diverse populations, a workshop participant suggested. However, the participant continued, it is not clear at this time whether it might be possible to convince policy makers to include genomic testing as one of the essential health benefits that insurance plans must cover. Genomic testing is not yet at a cost point that it would be feasible to develop and implement such a policy, Leonard said. It might be more realistic to consider at some point in the future—after genomic testing has been implemented in certain settings and if there is research demonstrating the long-term usefulness of genomic testing across a population. Korf agreed and said the field is currently in evidence-generating mode. Data being collected now will be the basis for such future policy decisions. The Alabama Genomic Health Initiative was funded by the policy makers in the state, and this demonstrates a real interest on their part in the potential application of genomic testing, Korf said. The evidence-generating process that resulted in the list of essential health benefits was based on the work of such groups as the U.S. Preventative Services Task Force and on recommendations from the National Academies and CDC, Isham said. It is important to consider the type of evidence cascade that will be needed to bring policy makers to a consensus about genomics as an essential health benefit in the future.

Participant and Public Engagement

The genomics-based programs described in the session had infrastructure built in for participant and public engagement, a workshop participant observed. She asked about the vision for conducting research to inform how programs engage with and consent different populations, given the different funding models and different contexts of the programs. The Alabama Genomic Health Initiative was envisioned as an opportunity to generate evidence, Korf said, as well as an opportunity to raise awareness and educate the public and providers about the growing field of genomics. There is a significant budget for education and outreach in the program, and there are a variety of engagement activities planned and under way. (For further discussion about participant engagement, see Chapter 5.) There is probably much more opportunity for data collection than there are resources to make the most use of the data at this time, Korf said.

---

[12]Essential health benefits are categories of services that health insurance plans must cover under the Patient Protection and Affordable Care Act. More information about the essential health benefits is available at https://www.healthcare.gov/glossary/essential-health-benefits (accessed February 14, 2018).

3

Financial Considerations for Implementing Genomics-Based Screening Programs

Highlights of Key Points Made by Individual Speakers

- While patients place a high value on the return of action-able genetic test findings, many also want to receive inciden-tal findings, regardless of treatability. *Personal utility* is the value that individuals receive from genomic information apart from health outcomes (i.e., the value of knowing), but this is not captured by traditional approaches to cost effectiveness. When this knowledge (i.e., personal utility) from the patient and public perspective is incorporated, it can lead to informed and successful financial investments on behalf of health care systems and individuals. (Peterson, Regier)
- Given the limited size of the currently available genetic coun-seling workforce, it is not possible to provide pretest genetic counseling on a population level. Similarly, frontline clini-cians may need to explain pharmacogenomic results to their patients, as there are not enough counselors to provide infor-mation during the prescribing process. (Peterson, Powell)
- When the prevalence of a genetic condition or disease is low in the general population, the number of false positive screening results can be greater than the number of true positive results, even with an assay that is highly sensitive and specific. Even though the vast majority of individuals who are negative for a specific variant will appropriately screen negative, some will

> screen falsely positive and will receive medical care they do not need. This must be taken into account when designing a genomic screening program to ensure that the program will be cost effective. (Powell)

In this session, panelists considered the financial aspects of genomics-based programs, including demonstrating value and the return on investment of screening programs. Bradford Powell, an assistant professor in the Department of Genetics at the University of North Carolina at Chapel Hill, provided an overview of the economic issues related to the implementation of genomics-based screening programs. Josh Peterson, an associate professor of biomedical informatics and medicine at Vanderbilt University Medical Center, described two ongoing programs to illustrate the drivers of value for pharmacogenomics panel testing. Dean Regier, an assistant professor at the University of British Columbia, discussed the concept of personal utility from his perspective as a health economist.

CLINICAL COSTS AND EFFECTS OF GENOMIC SCREENING

The difference between diagnostic testing and screening becomes important when considering the potential value of a genomic test. *Diagnostic testing* is performed for an individual who either has or is suspected of having a particular disorder because of clinical symptoms, Powell said. The prior probability that the person has the condition is relatively high, and testing can inform treatment or expectations of prognosis. In contrast, Powell said, *screening* is a population-based method for identifying persons with a condition or predisposition to a condition when the prior probability of having that condition is low. Screening may "inflict" health care on apparently healthy individuals who might never become sick with whatever condition is being screened for, he said.

Opportunistic screening occurs when a patient comes to a clinic for specific testing (e.g., pharmacogenomic variant testing for warfarin) and is tested at the same time for several high-yield variants related to common complex diseases (e.g., familial hypercholesterolemia, hereditary breast and ovarian cancer, and Lynch syndrome). Although opportunistic screening itself has a relatively low marginal cost, Powell said, there are challenges with generalizing it to population-level screening. The American College of Medical Genetics and Genomics (ACMG) has suggested that providers who offer genomic screening should provide pretest counseling, and it has developed a list of highly actionable gene variants for which it recommends reporting of incidental findings (Green et al., 2013). However, Powell said, it is not possible to provide the same degree of pretest counseling on a

---

BOX 3-1
Wilson and Jungner Screening Criteria

Characteristics of the **condition**:
- An important health problem (reasonable prevalence)
- Well-understood natural history
- Recognizable latent or early symptomatic phase in which treatment is more effective
- Have an accepted treatment for patients with recognized disease

Characteristics of **case finding**:
- Based on a suitable test or examination (acceptable to the population)
- Economically balanced in terms of other health care expenditures
- A continuing process (not "once and for all")

Characteristics of the **system**:
- Available facilities for diagnosis and treatment
- Risks (physical and psychological) less than the benefits
- Costs balanced against the benefits

SOURCES: Bradford Powell, National Academies of Sciences, Engineering, and Medicine workshop presentation, November 1, 2017. Adapted from Wilson and Jungner, 1968.

---

population level with the currently available workforce. There are also questions about how the estimated penetrance of these mutations will hold up against the ascertainment bias under which they were initially described.

When considering screening for additional conditions with new technologies, it is worth revisiting the screening criteria developed by Wilson and Jungner (1968). Powell presented those criteria reorganized by the characteristics of the condition, the characteristics of the case finding, and the characteristics of the health care system (see Box 3-1). By weighing the criteria listed above, it is possible to determine if it makes sense to implement screening for a given condition.

When Should Genomic Screening Be Performed?

Screening is most effective when performed prior to the age at which a condition's symptoms are likely to appear or the age at which the earliest stage of treatment can begin, Powell said. Prenatal screening—or even preconception screening—might be maximally effective with regard to actionability, he said, as it creates the opportunity to inform reproductive decision making. Because of the ethical quandaries that come with newborn (or earlier) genomic screening, it has been suggested that certain conditions should not be screened for until adulthood. Powell explained that according to the current ethical framework within clinical genetics, in the case of conditions with adult onset or for which an intervention is not started until adulthood, screening should be deferred and the child's future autonomy maintained (Ross et al., 2013). However, screening for different conditions may be indicated at different times throughout a person's life, and the financial feasibility of screening for genomic information may be different at different points in time. One potential solution, Powell said, is to "sequence first and ask questions later," obtaining the genetic sequence that can then be queried over time. Taking this approach raises questions of how the costs would be handled (initially, and over time). For example, relatively low-risk individuals may not benefit from genomic screening for a long time, and, with the current health care system, payers do not have a long enough time horizon with a given patient to benefit financially from the screening.

When Should Results Be Returned?[1]

When considering genomic screening in children, the issue of genetic exceptionalism[2] becomes particularly relevant, Powell said. Genomic screening in children involves proxy decision making by the parents on behalf of the child. As mentioned above, there are concerns about preserving the child's future autonomy. Deferring screening for adult onset conditions is one approach, but some patients and stakeholders have pushed back on this, Powell said. Concerns expressed include: What if this is the only genomic screening the child gets? What if testing indicates the parent might be at risk for a treatable, adult onset condition (e.g., hereditary breast and ovarian cancer)?

The question of what results should be returned when healthy infants undergo genomic screening has been incorporated as part of the North Carolina Newborn Exome Sequencing for Universal Screening (NC Nexus) Study.[3] This is being done in a controlled environment because of the potential risks, including financial risks, that might be carried by the children

---

[1] The National Academies of Sciences, Engineering, and Medicine has convened a committee to examine the return of individual-specific research results generated in research laboratories. For more information about the committee and consensus study, see http://nationalacademies. org/hmd/Activities/Research/ResearchResultsGeneratedinResearchLaboratories.aspx (accessed January 18, 2018).

[2] *Genetic exceptionalism* is the concept that genetic information should be treated differently than other medical information and deserves special privacy protections (Rothstein, 2005).

[3] For more information about the NC Nexus Study, see https://www.med.unc.edu/genetics/ berglab/Research/nc-nexus-project (accessed January 18, 2018).

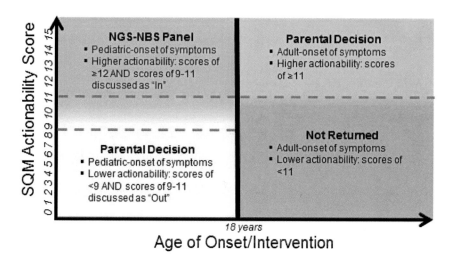

FIGURE 3-1 Considerations with regard to the return of genomic screening results performed on infants.
NOTE: NGS-NBS = next-generation sequencing–newborn screening; SQM = semi-quantitative metric.
SOURCE: Bradford Powell, National Academies of Sciences, Engineering, and Medicine workshop presentation, November 1, 2017.

over their lifetimes, Powell said. For a given childhood condition or gene variant, the actionability score (a semi-quantitative metric that weighs the severity of the disease, the likelihood of the outcome, the efficacy of a given intervention, the acceptability of the intervention, and the knowledge base supporting the disease and intervention [Powell, 2016]) is considered relative to the age of onset or intervention of the condition (see Figure 3-1). If a result is considered to be actionable within childhood, that condition/gene variant could potentially be included in a next-generation genomic sequencing newborn screening panel. Another part of the study randomizes parents into two groups which are then asked to decide whether they want to receive genomic screening information: those parents whose child screens positive for a pediatric-onset condition with a low actionability score, and those whose child screens positive for an adult-onset condition with a higher actionability score.[4]

---

[4]For more information about parental decision making about newborn genomic screening, see http://pediatrics.aappublications.org/content/137/Supplement_1/S16 (accessed January 18, 2018).

Genomic screening in adults involves different issues, in part because adults make their own decisions. The GeneScreen project[5] at the University of North Carolina at Chapel Hill is looking at the best ways to provide genomic screening to the general adult population. The study is designed to screen for a smaller subset of genes that are expected to provide the majority of health benefits across the population (including 17 genes for 11 conditions), Powell said, noting that when analyzing the results of the study, it will be important to take into account the fact that the prevalence of these individual conditions is low and there are concerns about the false discovery rate. The most common conditions among the 59 medically actionable genes listed by the ACMG have incomplete penetrance, Powell added. When prevalence is low in the general population, the number of false positive results can be greater than the number of true positive results. For example, if a condition is present in 1 in 10,000 individuals, and the screening test is 99 percent sensitive and 99.94 percent specific, it would be expected to find 699 positive screens in 1 million people. One hundred people will actually have the condition, and the sensitivity of the assay means that of those people, 99 will have a positive result, and 1 person will have a false negative result. Even though this is a very specific screen, and the vast majority of the 999,900 individuals who are negative will appropriately screen negative, 600 negative individuals will screen falsely positive (i.e., for each true positive result, there will be 6 false positives). Those individuals will receive medical care that they do not need.

For metabolic conditions in the newborn screen (e.g., phenylketonuria), secondary testing is performed to confirm positive results before any intervention. However, such secondary testing is not possible for many of the conditions that might be considered for a genomic screening panel, Powell said. Importantly, when "likely pathogenic" screening results have a 90 to 95 percent probability of being truly pathogenic, the screen is identifying people who would not have needed treatment (Plon et al., 2008; Richards et al., 2015).

Who Pays and Who Benefits?

Because health care in the United States uses a third-party payer system, there are different potential incentives to participate in genomic screening programs. Ideally, genomic screening programs should result in better patient care. There are also potential conflicts of interest to keep in mind, Powell said. For example, leaders at a health care system might be interested in identifying people at risk for colon cancer because the health care

---

[5]For more information about the GeneScreen project, see http://genomics.unc.edu/genomics andsociety/GeneScreen.html (accessed January 24, 2018).

system may benefit from performing additional colonoscopies. A pharmaceutical company might benefit from individuals being identified as being at higher risk for a certain side effect because those individuals might be prescribed a more costly agent. Whether these actions have a net benefit to patients or society depends on the prevalence of the condition and on how severe or frequent the adverse reaction would be, Powell said.

Drivers of Cost

There are three elements that drive the overall cost of genomic testing, Powell said: direct costs, downstream costs, and ancillary costs. At this stage, there are many hypotheses about the utility and applicability of genomic testing, but not enough data. Of the three types of costs, the direct costs (which include the cost of assays, analysis, and return of results) are the best characterized to date, although the cost of returning results is likely to change as current genomic screening efforts expand to population-level screening. Downstream costs include provider education, confirmatory testing, interventions and surveillance, and complications of interventions or surveillance. Ancillary costs include false reassurance (misunderstanding of information which may lead to people not seeking indicated care), interventions or surveillance in response to clinical false positive screens, patient anxiety or discomfort, and effects on insurance or employment. Powell noted that these ancillary costs can be quantified as quality-adjusted life years (QALYs) for comparison across different potential interventions.

Unknowns

There are still unknowns to be clarified before the balance of costs and benefits can be fully understood, Powell said. Unknowns include the prevalence of the conditions (the proportion of a population that has—or had—a specific condition in a given time period) (NIMH, 2017); the penetrance of the conditions (the percentage of individuals with a given genotype who exhibit the phenotype associated with that genotype) (Griffiths et al., 2000); and the efficacy of pre-symptomatic intervention, that is, how much of a difference identifying people at risk really makes. Until these variables are better characterized for each condition, there is a risk of treating people that do not need treatment, Powell said. In closing, he stressed the importance of being transparent and making sure that the patients and populations served by health care systems fully understand when screening is used to further research and when it is intended for clinical testing.

THE VALUE OF PHARMACOGENOMIC PANEL TESTING

To illustrate the drivers of value for pharmacogenomics panel testing, Peterson described two Vanderbilt University programs, a pharmacogenomic screening program integrated with the electronic health record (EHR) system called the Pharmacogenomic Resource for Enhanced Decisions in Care Treatment (PREDICT)[6] and an accompanying cost-effectiveness study designed to determine the long-term value of pharmacogenomic panel testing, Rational Integration of Genomic Healthcare Technology (RIGHT).[7]

Multiplex Pharmacogenomic Screening Panel

The typical testing approach at Vanderbilt University Medical Center has been evolving from serial, single gene testing to multiplexed panel testing. Multiplexed panels offer economies of scale, Peterson said, and the cost of assaying additional genetic variants approaches zero. Panels also broaden the opportunities to perform testing: preemptive screening (before clinically indicated) becomes feasible as well as reactive testing. Importantly, with preemptive testing clinicians do not need to remember to order each individual genetic test since the results of the panel are embedded in the EHR. This was one of the drivers of institutional investment in this area, Peterson said. On the other hand, he continued, clinicians may not want the responsibility of dealing with the additional patient data from pharmacogenomics testing. There is some additional cost associated with panel testing, both for the assay itself and for data management downstream, and any benefits are accrued in the future (when the test will presumably be cheaper and better). Peterson also noted that the genetic data might never be used if patients are not prescribed a relevant medication. There is also concern, especially by payers, about unintended or unwarranted costs related to cascade testing.

Common clinical scenarios motivated Vanderbilt's program for multiplexed pharmacogenomics screening, Peterson said; that program is integrated with the EHR as a way to provide opportunities to use a patient's genomic data over time. For example, a patient in the health system who has risk factors for coronary disease can be preemptively screened with the panel test and the results saved in his or her EHR. Later, if the patient develops coronary artery disease, he or she might receive percutaneous coronary intervention (a stent) and be prescribed antiplatelet therapy and statin therapy, which can be tailored according to the pharmacogenomic information in the EHR. Perhaps years later, the patient might develop

---

[6]For more information about PREDICT, see https://www.mydruggenome.org (accessed January 17, 2018).

[7]For more information about RIGHT, see http://rightsim.org or http://www.nber.org/papers/w24134 (accessed January 22, 2018).

atrial fibrillation and need anticoagulants, which can again be informed by the pharmacogenomic data.

Patients can enter the Vanderbilt PREDICT program through targeted preemptive screening or as a result of reactive testing. Preemptive screening is not reimbursed by payers, Peterson said, and the institution must cover the costs. In the case of reactive testing, there is a clinical indication and an ICD-9 code that can be used for billing purposes, and payers will cover the costs of at least one of the components on the panel. Once a patient is genotyped, the results are entered into the EHR, which includes clinical decision support for identified genetic risk variants. An example of using this information is the best practice alert, which interrupts the e-prescribing process and alerts the prescriber that the patient has a gene variant associated with an adverse reaction or variability of response for the drug being prescribed. The alert also includes recommendations for treatment modifications.

PREDICT relies on frontline clinicians to explain pharmacogenomic test results to their patients; however, there are not enough genetic counselors to be able to intervene with everyone during the prescribing process, Peterson said. To help with this, patients are also informed of their pharmacogenomic results through the patient portal, which provides high-level information about their pharmacogenetic test results and about how their genes affect their medications.

Determining the Value of Pharmacogenomic Testing

There are several lessons that have informed the economic modeling of pharmacogenomic screening, Peterson said.

- **Cost is a concern.** Cost does matter to clinicians, especially the expectation of reimbursement and the out-of-pocket costs for the patients they care for. There is also concern about the overall cost to the health system for something that is new and relatively unfamiliar.
- **Strength of evidence and guidelines matter.** Providers are particularly interested in guidelines from their clinical specialty. Guidelines from genetic societies have not yet been incorporated into guidelines from other specialties.
- **Clinical behavior is diverse.** Pharmacogenomic screening data are not deterministic. There are many reasons why providers might not follow the advice in the EHR alert. However, retrospective analysis shows that pharmacogenomic data do change prescribing substantially, with between 30 and 60 percent of prescriptions modified based on variants reported (Peterson et al., 2016).

Discrete event simulation is used to model indication (how often pharmacogenomic data would be used) and outcome (what the benefit of using those data would be), comparing genotyped and non-genotyped populations.[8] Peterson's group at Vanderbilt has created a model that incorporates all 46 drug–gene interactions on the level A list compiled by the Clinical Pharmacogenetics Implementation Consortium (CPIC).[9] To fully model cost effectiveness, Peterson said, it would be necessary to create a model for each individual interaction—all 46 of them. To simplify the simulation, the interactions were grouped into 7 categories according to frequency of prescribing, frequency of the adverse event, and severity of the adverse event, and 7 different models were created instead of 46.

In a simple genotype-tailored therapy model, Peterson explained, simulated patients receive the primary treatment or an alternate treatment, based on genotyping results. As in a real-life scenario, a certain number of adverse events are expected with the primary treatment. The simulated patients are followed through their lifetimes to death. The model relies on several base assumptions: that pharmacogenomics-guided therapy costs threefold more; pharmacogenomics guidance conveys 0.70 relative risk of adverse events; if not preemptively screened, a genetic test is ordered 50 percent of the time; and any genetic information obtained upstream is used 75 percent of the time. These are optimistic assumptions, Peterson said, and the simulation is run millions of times to determine what is driving the economic results.

Different strategies (no genotyping, reactive serial single-gene sequencing, preemptive panel, and reactive panel) have different likelihoods of being cost effective, given a certain willingness to pay for an extra QALY, Peterson said. Figure 3-2 depicts the projected likelihood for each scenario. An example of a procedure with a very high incremental cost-effectiveness ratio (ICER) is a left ventricular assist device, where the ICER exceeds $500,000; an example of a low incremental cost-effectiveness ratio is a colonoscopy, where patients gain an extra QALY for every $25,000 spent on the intervention. In this analysis, preemptive genotyping has a 50 percent chance of being cost effective relative to a willingness to pay of $150,000, although many groups set willingness to pay thresholds at $50,000 or $100,000, Peterson shared. Reactive serial single-gene testing

---

[8]For more detailed information, see "The Value of Genomic Pharmacogenomic Information," a working paper to be included in a forthcoming conference proceedings of the National Bureau of Economic Research. Available at http://www.nber.org/chapters/c13989 (accessed January 3, 2018).

[9]CPIC Level A indicates that genetic information should be used to change prescribing of an affected drug. To be defined as CPIC Level A, the preponderance of evidence must be high or moderate in favor of changing prescribing. For more information about the level definitions for CPIC gene–drug pairs see https://cpicpgx.org/prioritization/#flowchart (accessed February 8, 2018).

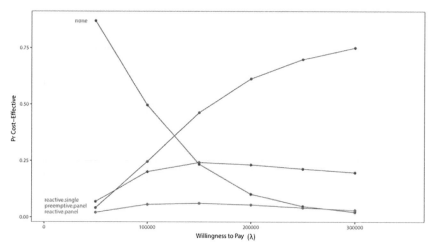

FIGURE 3-2 Projected likelihood of cost effectiveness.
NOTES: Pr = plausible range. Willingness to pay (x axis) is from the decision makers' perspective.
SOURCES: Joshua Peterson, National Academies of Sciences, Engineering, and Medicine workshop presentation, November 1, 2017. Originally from Graves et al., 2017.

is somewhat cost effective at the low end of willingness to pay, but cost effectiveness levels off and then decreases as willingness to pay increases. Reactive panel testing has a low probability of cost effectiveness across the spectrum of willingness to pay. A sensitivity analysis that plots the probability that pharmacogenomic information is used versus risk reduction from use of the pharmacogenomic-guided therapy is another way to analyze cost effectiveness of multiplexed testing strategies, Peterson said. If there is no reduction of the risk of an adverse event, then not testing is clearly preferred. If there is significant risk reduction, preemptive panel testing is the preferred option only if the probability that the clinician is going to use the data is high. If that probability is low, reactive single-gene testing is the better approach. Efforts to create implementation programs that are effective matter, Peterson said. As implementation approaches improve to a point where clinicians use pharmacogenomic data 100 percent of the time, preemptive panel testing becomes the optimal strategy.

Summary of Lessons Learned from the PREDICT Project

The key goals of the PREDICT project are to create a methodology with which to evaluate the use of pharmacogenomic information over a patient's lifetime and assess the value of panel testing. There are a number of assumptions under which multiplexed pharmacogenomic screening is cost effective, Peterson said, but the time frame for accrual of benefits to achieve cost effectiveness may be many years, especially in relatively low-risk individuals. In the current health care system, payers do not work under time horizons that are that long. The analyses conducted thus far are a traditional approach to cost effectiveness; there may be other kinds of value that are not being captured, such as the value of patients knowing their genomic test results and being confident in the safety and efficacy of the prescriptions, which can affect adherence and engagement in care.

COLORECTAL CANCER SCREENING AND RETURN OF SECONDARY FINDINGS: A VALUE FRAMEWORK ANALYSIS

The value-for-money approach considers costs relative to health outcomes, Regier said, describing the reference cases for estimating value for money used in Canada, the United Kingdom, and the United States. A reference case is used to lay out the principles and methods that are appropriate for particular institutional objectives. In Canada and the United Kingdom, the objective of the analysis is to maximize health status gains subject to limited budgets. To do this, an ICER is calculated by dividing the incremental cost by the QALY and then compared to how much the decision makers are willing to pay for each QALY gained. The reference case in Canada and the United Kingdom is the health system perspective—that is, the perspective of those who manage the budgets and need to meet the objective of maximum health gains across the population. The recently published guidance from the Second Panel on Cost Effectiveness in Health and Medicine for the United States takes this analysis a step further, calling for the inclusion of the societal perspective as well as the health care system perspective (Neumann et al., 2017). To achieve a societal perspective, researchers may want to go beyond standard analyses to consider broader costs and broader concepts of what patients value in their health care.

Regier explained that health economists typically estimate QALYs using the EQ5D questionnaire, a standardized tool created by the EuroQol group for measuring health status. The EQ5D consists of a set of questions that asks patients to rate their quality of life in five domains: mobility, self-care, usual activities, pain/discomfort, and anxiety/depression. In the EQ-5D-3L, each dimension has three possible responses that indicate whether the patient has no problems, some/moderate difficulties, or extreme difficulties/

incapacity in that dimension. These results are then calculated to inform the QALY, whose value lies between one, which is perfect health, and zero, which is death.[10]

Traditional measures of value and value for money in health economics are somewhat limited in their application to precision medicine and genomic technologies, Regier said. The value of precision medicine is dependent on the information that patients receive and the benefits that patients and providers ascribe to that information (Marshall et al., 2017). The Second Panel on Cost Effectiveness in Health and Medicine said that decision makers need a "quantification and valuation of all health and non-health effects of interventions, and to summarize those effects in a single quantitative measure" (Neumann et al., 2017, p. 370). The EQ5D estimate of QALY does not incorporate those non-health effects, Regier noted.

The Value of Knowing: Incorporating Preference-Based Utility

Regier said that from his perspective as an economist, value equals preference-based utility. In other words, the preferences of the individuals making decisions among alternative health care goods can inform the value of those goods. For precision medicine and genomics, Grosse and colleagues have said that personal utility is the utility that individuals and families ascribe to genomic information apart from health outcomes (Grosse et al., 2010). Personal utility enhances one's sense of control, informs self-identity, and can resolve uncertainties surrounding an individual's diagnosis and prognosis (Foster et al., 2009; Regier et al., 2009). The valuation of personal utility, Regier said, can be done using the stated preference discrete choice experiment method, which is based on an attribute-based measure of value that is based on random utility theory (McFadden, 1974). A discrete choice experiment is a well-established way of eliciting preferences for non-market health care products and programs and determining how individuals value various health states (Lancsar and Louviere, 2008).

Next-generation sequencing and secondary findings provide information on diseases that are not related to a patient's current diagnosis, Regier said. For example, a patient might be tested for Lynch syndrome, with the secondary findings indicating a risk for long QT syndrome (which is treatable) and Alzheimer's disease (for which there is no effective treatment). As discussed earlier in the day, the ACMG recommends the return of highly penetrant, clinically actionable results, without patient preference being fully taken into account; however, Regier said, the ACMG did not ask individuals what kind of information they wanted. In contrast, the Cana-

---

[10]For more information about the EQ5D and the EuroQol Group, see https://euroqol.org/eq-5d-instruments (accessed January 18, 2018).

dian College of Medical Genetics does not endorse returning actionable secondary findings for monogenic conditions outside of the research context because of the high cost, both psychological and monetary.

In a discrete choice experiment, Regier and colleagues asked a representative population of 1,200 Canadians what kind of information they wanted from secondary findings, if such information could be provided (Regier et al., 2015). Participants were presented with a series of exercises, and each time they were asked to choose between two scenarios for receiving information that differed with regard to disease risk, treatability, severity, carrier status, and cost to the patient. An econometric behavioral model was used to predict preference-based utility, which informed the uptake of different policy scenarios for the return of results and individuals' willingness to pay for the return of incidental findings. Willingness to pay is a measure of value, Regier clarified, and it is estimated as the monetary equivalent of preference-based utility. The results of the experiment showed that the Canadian population that had been surveyed valued secondary genomic information regardless of whether the condition was treatable. Participants decidedly wanted to have actionable findings returned, Regier said, but they also wanted to receive incidental findings regarding nontreatable conditions.

The cost effectiveness of returning secondary genomic findings was studied by Bennette and colleagues, who calculated the ICER (i.e., the incremental cost per QALY gain) (Bennette et al., 2015). Analyzing hypothetical cohorts of cardiomyopathy and colorectal cancer patients as well as the general population, they found that the ICER for return of secondary findings varied depending on the specific patient population. A key aspect of this analysis, Regier said, is decision uncertainty, which is the level of confidence that the ICER will fall below a certain willingness to pay for a QALY gain. There are some limits to this quantitative model, Regier said, in that there is no allowance for personal utility because it is not incorporated into the QALY metric. In addition, the analysis begins at the stage of return (or not) of secondary findings, and upstream costs and consequences are not examined.

Regier explained how he adapted Bennette and colleagues' model (Bennette et al., 2015) to answer questions about the cost effectiveness of genomic screening for colorectal cancer and polyposis (CRCP) syndromes and the return of secondary findings. By incorporating an allowance for personal utility (i.e., the value of knowing), Regier adapted the ICER equation to calculate net monetary benefit and include personal utility using willingness to pay. His model projected life expectancy and costs for two trajectories: one for an individual who received standard care for CRCP, and another for an individual who received a genomic screening panel and was given the secondary findings. For the latter trajectory, life expectancy and costs were also projected for relatives who were offered—and accepted or declined—genetic counseling and genetic testing. These models are data intensive, Regier said. Overall, the results suggest that the possible return of secondary findings was likely to be cost effective; however, he noted that there is a lot of decision uncertainty. When using the reference case for the United Kingdom and Canada (which does not factor in personal utility), Regier finds that the probability that CRCP screening and the return of secondary findings is cost effective to be 72 percent, which may be too much uncertainty for the typical decision maker in Canada or the United Kingdom, he said. When the concepts of personal utility and net benefit were incorporated, decision uncertainty was reduced. The probability that CRCP screening and the return of secondary findings was cost effective was 82 percent. Sequencing in Canada is currently fairly expensive, Regier said. The monetary cost of the hypothetical panel was calculated to be $4,600. Further analysis suggested that the probability of cost effectiveness (incorporating personal utility) could be increased to 95 percent if the hypothetical cost of the genomic screening panel and analysis was $3,200.

Considering Personal Utility and the Potential Value of Genomic Knowledge

Current guidelines for assessing the value of genomics technologies do not support the inclusion of personal utility, Regier concluded. However, when the value of precision medicine knowledge from the patient and public perspective is not incorporated, it can lead to the wrong investments by health care delivery systems (over-investment if patients have disutility for the knowledge of their own genomic variants; under-investment if patients place value on that knowledge). The proposed value framework allows for a broader analysis of value, beyond QALY.

From an applied perspective, Regier said, both upstream and downstream considerations are critical. In the absence of personal utility, decision uncertainty is quite substantial. Precision medicine and genomic technologies amplify already complex decisions regarding screening. Additional data are needed to support these complex decisions, including information from patients and the public regarding their perceptions of the value of personal genomic knowledge.

DISCUSSION

Data for Demonstrating Value

Data on penetrance is incredibly important, Powell said, describing which data he would prioritize to demonstrate the value of genomic testing.

As a clinician returning genomic results, he said, he wants to be able to give patients a sense of what they can expect based on the findings. Data sharing about drug response phenotypes across a large population is needed, Peterson added. Genotype information is often accessible, while phenotype data are more difficult to ascertain from the EHR. It will also be important, Regier said, to do a better job of engaging with patients and the public in order to develop an improved understanding of how they value different types of information and health outcomes.

While very large randomized controlled trials are ideal for demonstrating value to payers and guideline writers, some of the simulations conducted required analyzing millions of patients with certain characteristics to achieve the necessary precision, Peterson said, highlighting the need for improved methods for comparative effectiveness research with outside cohorts. There is also a need for better methods to understand cost effectiveness, Regier added. Randomized controlled trials in precision medicine will not be common or broad in scale.

Perspectives on Costs

It was observed that the costs of conducting panel-based preemptive testing are likely to vary over time, and a workshop participant asked how reductions in the cost of testing influence overall cost effectiveness and who bears these costs. Peterson replied that for a high-risk group that is likely to use the information right away, the cost of testing will be swamped by the cost of outcomes. In modeling the value of genomic information for tailoring antiplatelet therapy in coronary patients, for example, the cost of the test, which is generally modeled at $100 to $200, does not have a major influence on the overall economic output. The value proposition changes, however, when screening a very large, average-risk population. The cost of doing business in this area should be split between health care systems, which might indirectly accrue a lot of value for this kind of work, and insurers, who also have a stake, Peterson suggested. From a health care system point of view, there are costs which will not be directly covered by insurers, such as the costs of data management, data, or staff time for delivering information to clinicians or assisting with decision making. These types of costs are difficult to incorporate into the cost of the actual assay. Assay cost is a moving target, Regier agreed, noting the Personalized Oncogenomics Program at the Genome Sciences Center in British Columbia does whole-genome transcriptome analysis for patients with incurable cancers and uses forecasting methods to help understand where that moving target might go in the future.

Most large employers are self-insured and use payers as a third-party administrator, a workshop participant said. It is then the employer who is responsible for determining health care benefits, along with other employee benefits. The participant asked if cost–benefit and return on investment from an employer's perspective were different from an insurance company perspective and if health economists model from an employer's perspective, noting that employee recruitment, retention, and return on investment for some industry sectors and employers can be modeled over 10 years, instead of 1 or 2 years for an insurance member relationship. There are many different people involved in making those decisions, with many different competing interests. Personal utility, for example, is not going to be important to an insurance company, Powell said. It may, however, be important to an employer, because an employer will design benefits and health care coverage to try to attract and retain the desired workforce. Economic analyses can be done from many different perspectives, Veenstra added. It was suggested that when seeking to convince payers to adopt the routine reimbursement of genomics, forward-thinking employers might be more successful targets than a large insurance company or the Centers for Medicare & Medicaid Services. Potential models should emphasize the employer's perspective, rather than other payer perspectives.

Pharmacist Role in Pharmacogenomics

Clinical pharmacists are critical for clinical decision support, Peterson said, and most hospitals have pharmacists who are assigned to specific teams (e.g., a transplant pharmacist). Unfortunately, the prescribing alert in the EHR is not pushed out to all of the systems that the pharmacists use. There are surveillance systems that the pharmacists use which run alongside the EHR and pick up pharmacogenomic information on current patients.

Taking Clinical Practice and Uptake into Account

There are challenges associated with accounting for clinical practice in models that use retrospective data, observed a workshop participant. For example, if a retrospective economic analysis shows a certain number of actionable variants but in practice only a portion of those are actually being acted on, how can that information be accounted for in the economic analysis? How can the message be delivered to providers that improvement in clinical practice to achieve optimal use, or even appropriate use, could provide a greater cost effectiveness? The behavior of physicians and patients is an extremely important aspect, Peterson agreed, noting that one of the aims of his study is to examine how such behavior influences economic outcomes. The more likely it is that the incidental data are used, the more likely the patient is to benefit from having preemptive screening.

Economic models can vary widely depending on uptake (whether the patient wants the information, whether the clinician returns the result), Regier added. If decision models are done well (and they are often not), they will incorporate uptake into the model as a probability, he said. The difficulty comes when a novel technology is involved and the degree of uptake is not known. The challenge then is to predict uptake (i.e., patient and clinician preferences) in a way that has external validity, he said, noting that this is what the discrete choice experiment is meant to do. Incomplete uptake leads to varying budget impacts across the health care system. There are advanced techniques—referred to by the general term "value of information analysis"—that can be used to compare the value of doing more research versus the value of getting things implemented, Veenstra said. Such analyses can help to structure these issues and identify evidence gaps.

Incorporating the Heterogeneity of Personal Utility Preferences

It is important to take diversity and diverse populations into account when collecting information on how the general population values genome screening and results. There is no "average patient," Regier said, and the challenge is how to incorporate the heterogeneity of value or preferences. There are methods being developed that are starting to address this. In the Canadian population he sampled, for example, there was a range of age representation, jurisdictional representation across the provinces, and representation across languages. One population that was missing, however, was Aboriginal First Nations representation, and there is a gap in understanding value among those in traditionally underserved communities.

Information about diverse individuals is often lacking at the biological level as well, and the understanding of founder variants and benign population variants is limited, Powell added. There is also the potential to exacerbate economic disparities with genomic screening. For example, identifying a condition that a person cannot get treatment for can cause more harm than benefit for that person.

There is variation by geography as well as by socioeconomic status, observed a workshop participant. Health literacy and economic and educational factors vary in populations and affect personal utility. Socioeconomic status, including income, geography, and age, affect preferences and personal utility, Regier agreed. Better communication and decision aids are needed to help people make very complex decisions about what information they want. There is an opportunity to engage with patients and the public and provide them with some level of genomic literacy (e.g., explaining terms such as penetrance, treatability, and clinical utility) so these individuals can have conversations with their providers and choose the options that are consistent with the underlying value of the information for them.

Opportunistic Screening

Feero raised the issue of opportunistic approaches to screening (i.e., testing for an additional set of variants when sequencing is ordered for a specific clinical question). By implementing opportunistic screening, relevant genomic data on larger segments of the population are slowly being accrued. Once there has been a commitment to conduct the original genomic test, the incremental cost for adding several additional tests would seem to be quite small, Feero said.

Decision Tools

It is challenging for providers to determine which panel will provide the most benefit for the patient from the many different panels available, a workshop participant commented. Developing decision tools for clinicians to help select the most appropriate panel from what is available may help providers identify the best panel, the participant suggested. There are ongoing efforts to develop decision aids, Peterson said, but unfortunately there is wide variability in terms of how those decision algorithms work or even what variants are on the panel. In his practice, he said, he prefers to work with companies and panels that are transparent in terms of both what is on the panel and how the company uses it to arrive at a recommendation. There are also guidelines that reflect academic agreement on how a particular variant should be used in clinical practice.

There is a risk of creating panels that are so broad that they include variants for which there is not sufficient evidence of utility, Powell added. Such testing creates the risk of doing research under the guise of clinical testing. Projects such as ClinGen will help increase understanding of the genes and the variants for which there is sufficient information to make recommendations for screening, but there is a need to be clear about what testing is research, he said. Different panels are used in different health care systems in Canada, Regier said, and some health care systems do not have access to any genomic panel testing, raising the issue of equity across the country.

Considering Ways to Move Forward

To inform the Roundtable's development of activities, Ginsburg asked the panel what the population health community should be doing to accelerate the types of modeling discussed and to provide information to institutional decision makers who are considering implementing genomics-based programs. Costs change rapidly over time, Peterson said. While there is value to knowing the current costs, the 5- to 10-year value of the work being done now will be reliant on the clinical outcomes. The models show that outcomes drive costs, and, from a societal health care perspective, achieving the best possible clinical outcome is the priority, he said. A standardized cost can be attached to that clinical outcome, which has some transferability across health care systems. There is a movement toward embedding health economics within many genome-scale sequencing projects, Powell said, adding that this movement should be encouraged and mentioning the National Human Genome Research Institute's Ethical, Legal and Social Implications Research Program. It is important to engage budgetary decision makers and provide them with reliable but not overly complicated information, Regier suggested, noting that health economists often present information at a level that is too technically complex. There is also a need to bring the public and patients into the conversations around value, he concluded.

4

Exploring Approaches to Optimize Data Sharing Among Early Implementers of Genomics-Based Programs

---

Highlights of Key Points Made by Individual Speakers

- Sharing by researchers and project managers should go beyond genomic data to the sharing of experiences, methods, and phenotypic data from the electronic health record. Common data models and data standards can help facilitate improved data sharing. (Chisholm, Grodman, Orlando)
- An analysis commons brings data (genomic and phenotypic) and resources (analytical tools) in proximity in a secure environment and makes them available to authorized users for the purpose of accelerating translation and promoting further discovery. (Boerwinkle)
- When evaluating the clinical utility of a genomics-based trial or program, it is important to evaluate common functional genotypes that are pertinent to the specific patient population(s) under study to avoid systematic misclassification of variant carriers as wild-type. (Turner)[a]
- For pharmacogenomic implementation studies, guideline adherence by practitioners and adherence to prescribed medications by patients are important outcomes to measure, and systems should be designed to record this information. (Turner)

---

[a]This highlight was revised after the prepublication release.

- Incentives for collaboration and data sharing can include securing funding, improving statistical power (especially for demonstrating clinical utility and cost effectiveness), enhancing the recruitment of research participants, facilitating economies of scale, mitigating risk, and developing shared solutions (e.g., streamlined ethical approvals). (Turner)
- Implementation efforts need structure as a way to provide guidance on future efforts in other settings and to provide a model for the development of sustainability. (Orlando)
- Patients will drive the demand for data sharing as they become the gatekeepers of their medical record data. (Boerwinkle, Chisholm)

Various different models for integrating genomic testing into health care systems were discussed at the workshop, but there is not a one-size-fits-all approach, said session moderator Marc Grodman, an assistant professor of clinical medicine at Columbia University. The genomics-based programs under discussion at this workshop test for different genetic variants, are performed by different people, and are being paid for through different mechanisms. Out of these many programs volumes of data are being generated, and there are challenges to sharing those data both within and across institutions and systems. Furthermore, Grodman said, sharing goes beyond the sharing of data to the sharing of experiences, methods, and approaches. Panelists in this session discussed approaches to information sharing across systems and organizations. Rex Chisholm, the vice dean for scientific affairs and graduate education at Northwestern University, described the Electronic Medical Records and Genomics (eMERGE) network as an example of sharing data across a consortium and linking genotypic information to the electronic health record (EHR). Eric Boerwinkle, the dean and M. David Low Chair in Public Health at the University of Texas Health Science Center at Houston, discussed optimizing the sharing of data, results, experiences, and resources. Richard Turner, a clinical research fellow in clinical pharmacology and therapeutics at the Royal Liverpool University Hospital and the University of Liverpool, described some of the incentives and challenges of data sharing in three implementation projects in Europe. Lori Orlando, an associate professor of medicine at Duke University School of Medicine, discussed the importance of applying implementation science when launching genomics-based programs, including defining and developing measures for genomic medicine implementation studies.

DATA SHARING LESSONS FROM THE EMERGE NETWORK

The eMERGE network[1] is a National Human Genome Research Institute (NHGRI)-funded consortium consisting of nine active clinical sites, two sequencing centers, and a coordinating center, explained Chisholm, who is one of the principal investigators of eMERGE. The goal of the eMERGE network is to combine DNA repositories with EHR systems for large-scale, high-throughput genetic research that supports the implementation of genomic medicine. Peterson is the principal investigator of the coordinating center at Vanderbilt University, Chisholm said, and what has been done across the sites in the eMERGE network is a microcosm of what will need to be done in rolling out genomic medicine across the country.

eMERGE is a rich resource, Chisholm said, with genome-wide association studies data from over 100,000 participants to date. Genetic data from individuals at eMERGE sites are merged with their EHRs and used for genomic research. This linking of genotypic information to the EHR allows for very efficient use of the data, Chisholm said, and as part of the group's efforts 84 important genes for drug metabolism have been sequenced in more than 9,000 participants. The commitment to enter that information in the EHRs and to use it to inform clinical decision support enables the assessment of the value of pharmacogenomics in a clinical setting, he said. eMERGE is currently recruiting 25,000 additional participants who will have a gene panel of 109 genes sequenced. These will include the 59 genes identified as medically actionable by the American College of Medical Genetics and Genomics, other genes of interest to the research project, and numerous single nucleotide polymorphisms, many of which are relevant to pharmacogenomics (Kalia et al., 2017). The clinical sequencing centers will then return actionable data to the EHRs.

In this system, data are transferred from the clinical sequencing centers to the clinical sites. Previously the sequencing center associated with eMERGE would send genomic data to the clinical site in a portable document format (i.e., as PDF files); however, Chisholm said, now the network is able to get an XML feed of the data, which allows for greater interoperability. Building on that accomplishment and continuing to establish data exchange standards would help facilitate the exchange of data, he said.

Sharing Data to Support Value Measurement

Data sharing can enable more robust and meaningful results, Chisholm said. The data from any one clinical site alone are unlikely to provide the

---

[1]For more information on the eMERGE network, see https://www.genome.gov/27540473/electronic-medical-records-and-genomics-emerge-network (accessed January 10, 2018).

statistical power to draw meaningful conclusions regarding value. However, a cohort of more than 100,000 people like those in the eMERGE network offers increased statistical power to study many common diseases.

The use of data standards is important for data sharing, Chisholm continued. The meaningfulness of combining data together in one place is limited if systems are using different languages to collect those data. By using common data models and common standards, eMERGE has been able to facilitate data sharing. eMERGE participants are now working to convert all of the data to the Observational Medical Outcomes Partnership (OMOP) common data model,[2] which will be instrumental in improving data sharing going forward, Chisholm said. The OMOP common data model allows for systematic analyses of disparate observational databases.

The sharing of phenotypic data from EHRs also presents unique challenges, and eMERGE has adopted a hybrid model with data standards to address this issue. eMERGE shares a collection of phenotypic data (mostly coded data) with the coordinating center, which makes it available through the eRecordCounter tool. This tool allows researchers to ask a specific question of the records, such as, How many people are there with type II diabetes and a body mass index over 40 who are not taking insulin? Exploratory data figures are then shared with researchers to help them with project planning and feasibility assessment.

Overcoming Obstacles to Data Sharing

When the eMERGE network began, one of the first processes was to develop a data use agreement outlining the principles for data sharing. The first attempt at drafting a data use agreement included legal language from the five initial sites in the consortium, and the result was a massive document that was not helpful to most stakeholders, Chisholm said. The process started over with a simple draft and a focus on what the consortium was trying to accomplish. eMERGE leadership worked with each site's principal investigators and lawyers and explained the process and the need for a simple agreement. What developed was a standardized data use agreement that did not have a lot of extra language, and when additional sites joined the consortium, the agreement could be signed without the need for any changes.

As mentioned, one of the technological barriers to data sharing is a lack of data standards. When eMERGE began, Chisholm said, concerns were raised about using clinical data for research purposes. It was found, however, that there is value in using clinical data in a repeated, regular

---

[2] For more information about the OMOP common data model, see https://www.ohdsi.org/data-standardization/the-common-data-model (accessed January 10, 2018).

way and that doing so can actually improve the quality of data for clinical care. As an example, Chisholm said, an initial analysis of birthweight in an obstetrics hospital with 13,000 deliveries each year revealed an odd bimodal distribution, which led to the realization that some entries were in grams, while others were in kilograms. Simply constraining the numbers that could be entered immediately led to an improvement in the data quality in the EHRs. Deploying standards that are shared across a variety of organizations is beneficial across health care and certainly for precision medicine and genomic medicine approaches, he said.

Common Data Elements

There are many data elements, such as the reactions of participants and providers, that it would be helpful to collect to inform the implementation of genomics-based programs. In implementing pharmacogenomics at Northwestern, Chisholm said, a lot of communication and training was required in order to demonstrate to primary care providers that there is value in putting pharmacogenomic information into the EHR.

Information is also needed about health care use to inform economic discussions, Chisholm said. One barrier to implementing precision medicine broadly is the fear that that it will overwhelm the health care system with additional work that brings little value. It is important to capture the type of usage data discussed by Goddard (see Chapter 2) and to share it broadly across organizations, Chisholm said.

OPTIMIZING DATA SHARING

Health care is an integral and growing part of the U.S. economy, Boerwinkle said. However, sharing information is often thought of as counter to profitability because many chief financial officers in large health care systems view sharing as an avenue to lose patients from their system, he said. It is important to consider sharing more broadly and take advantage of new business models emerging around the "sharing economy." Boerwinkle suggested that patients drive the demand for data sharing as they take on the role of being gatekeepers for their medical record data.

As an example of sharing in a large, complex environment, Boerwinkle discussed optimizing the sharing of data, resources, and results and experience at the Texas Medical Center. The center includes 59 member institutions collectively logging 10 million patient visits each year. If the Texas Medical Center were to incorporate, he said, it would be the eighth largest economic zone in the country. As such, it is an ideal test bed for sharing data across health care systems.

Data Sharing: HealthConnect

Ideally a data sharing system would connect all health care providers. There is often a discussion about placing all health care data in the cloud so everyone can access it, Boerwinkle said, but this would not be the most efficient approach for health care or for research. There is also interest in health information exchanges (HIEs), which are quite effective in some parts of the country, he said. In an ideal HIE, all of the health care entities in the exchange share data in semi-real time, based on queries from any of the nodes. The entities include, for example, hospitals, radiology centers, pharmacies, clinics, laboratories, primary care providers, and specialists.

HealthConnect, a community master patient index, is used by the Texas Medical Center, Boerwinkle explained. The index receives real-time information about all patient visits and activity. Every individual in the health care system has a set of identifiers and can be mapped independently of the place where he or she is having a medical encounter. In practice, any one of the participating organizations (e.g., hospitals, health care systems) can make a data request to the HealthConnect system. In a matter of seconds, HealthConnect can confirm that a particular patient has consented to sharing his or her information, can locate information about that unique patient across the different organizations in the HealthConnect community, and can query a target organization if needed. Then, within hours, the target organization responds to the data query with additional information about the patient's medical care. In this way, competing health care systems are sharing data for the benefit of the patient, Boerwinkle said, without fear of losing patients to a competing system.

Optimizing Results and Experience Sharing: Standards of Evidence

The ClinGen project is a venue for sharing genomic information that includes the vetting of information by experts, developing standards, and moving toward actionability (Rehm et al., 2015). However, Boerwinkle said, scaling the approach of ClinGen will be challenging because of the need to establish the clinical validity of the variants with groups of experts. The ability to scale the sharing of genomic information is essential for genomics to become integrated into the routine health care setting. Developing semi-automated clinical reporting platforms and machine-learning algorithms to help with establishing the clinical validity of variants and matching variant characteristics to phenotypic characteristics may be one useful approach. Another possible approach, Boerwinkle said, is crowd-sourcing the curation of genomic data and the interpretation of variants in order to tap into the tremendous expertise in the health community.

Resource Sharing: Developing an Analysis Commons

The successful academic health care centers will be those that move their discoveries into the translational space and make those data and their translational experiences available to researchers for further discovery, Boerwinkle said. This will create a cycle of clinical care and research, leading to a learning health care system.

In terms of a resource for sharing research, he said that researchers are not generally going to the EHR for health data. Rather, health data are moved to a data warehouse, outside of the EHR, where researchers can mine the information. This calls for the creation of an environment that brings the data (genomic and phenotypic) and the analytical tools in proximity, in a secure analysis commons. The data in the commons would be made available to authorized users, after appropriate vetting. DNAnexus is one example of an analysis platform that can be accessed by the research community, Boerwinkle said.

IMPLEMENTING PHARMACOGENOMICS IN EUROPE

Ubiquitous Pharmacogenomics Consortium

Three ongoing initiatives in Europe can provide examples of the incentives and challenges of genomic data sharing, Turner said. The Ubiquitous Pharmacogenomics (U-PGx) consortium is a pan-European endeavor involving 16 beneficiaries across 10 European Union (EU) countries.[3] U-PGx is funded for 5 years by a Horizon 2020 grant through the European Commission. The centerpiece of the project, Turner said, is a 3-year pharmacogenomic implementation study occurring at one or more sites in seven EU countries, including the Royal Liverpool Hospital in the United Kingdom. The study will evaluate implementation metrics, patient outcomes, and cost effectiveness. Over the 3-year study period, 8,000 participants will be recruited to either a standard-of-care arm or a pharmacogenomic-tailored care arm in which they will be preemptively genotyped for 50 variants in 13 pharmacogenes. A guideline will be given to their care practitioners (who may or may not follow the dosing recommendation). Participants will be followed for a minimum of 12 weeks in order to identify adverse drug reactions. Turner noted that, due to the nature of the funding call, this is not a randomized controlled trial but rather an implementation study. The 3-year study period is divided into two 18-month blocks. For each participating country, one 18-month block will be designated to standard of care, and

---

[3]For more information regarding the Ubiquitous Pharmacogenomics consortium, see http://upgx.eu (accessed January 3, 2018).

the other block will be designated to pharmacogenomic-tailored care. The order of these two arms has been randomized across the seven countries.

Turner described a number of operational factors involved in getting the study up and running. In obtaining ethical approvals, the Netherlands and the United Kingdom were instrumental in first going to their organizing regulatory bodies to demonstrate that this is an implementation study and not a randomized controlled trial. This helped facilitate ethical approvals on a similar basis for most of the other partners, he said. Another factor was that the Dutch Pharmacogenetics Working Group's guidelines needed to be translated into the language of each participating country.[4] It is not just the language, but the cultural acceptability that must be considered in translation, Turner said. For example, in trying to capture quality-of-life information, time trade-off questions were not acceptable to patients in Italy or the United Kingdom, and the questionnaire needed to be revised accordingly. Interestingly, he said, time trade-off questions were more acceptable to people in Austria and the Netherlands.

One of the benefits of working together is economies of scale, Turner said. Genotyping is being performed locally at the seven sites, on the same platform. All of the information is then sent to bio.logis (a genetic information management firm in Frankfurt) to carry out standardized genotype interpretation. As new evidence is accrued, the bio.logis site is updated, and standardized information is automatically returned to the sites. In the United Kingdom, for example, the university is responsible for the study, patients are recruited from the Royal Liverpool Hospital, genotyping will be carried out in a clinically accredited laboratory, and data will be submitted to bio.logis and then fed back to both the hospital and the study case report form. One challenge, Turner said, is the wide spectrum of current standards within health care systems across the EU. Greece is generally paper based, while the Royal Liverpool Hospital is paperless. As such, it has been necessary to allow the sites the flexibility to develop ways to make the genetic information available to their practitioners. In the Netherlands and the United Kingdom, the plan is to have an interruptive clinical decision support system. At other sites, practitioners may simply receive a PDF document. In an auxiliary approach, the genetic information will be associated with a quick response (QR) code on a credit card–sized "Safety-Code" card held by the patient, and primary care practitioners can easily access the information by scanning the QR code using a smartphone.[5]

Turner listed several outcomes that should be measured in pharmacoge-

---

[4]For more information about the Dutch Pharmacogenetics Working Group, see https://www.pharmgkb.org/page/dpwg (accessed January 17, 2018).

[5]For more information on the Medication Safety Code System, see http://safety-code.org (accessed January 3, 2018).

nomic studies. For example, there is no mandate to follow the pharmacogenomic recommendations as part of this study, so it is important to look at guideline adherence by practitioners. Unfortunately, current systems are not designed to record this information. In addition, for pharmacogenomic studies it is important to take drug adherence into account. If a patient is not taking a prescribed drug, then the reasons for the non-adherence should be sought. Other outcomes to consider include surrogate markers, health care use and associated costs, prescription changes, clinical utility, and, ultimately, quality-of-life information.

Warfarin Pharmacogenomics Implementation

There are several factors that can affect the determination of clinical utility for genomics-based programs, including patient ethnicity, the baseline characteristics of the health care service, specific drug indications, and implementation knowledge and attitudes. Turner elaborated on these factors in the context of warfarin pharmacogenomics implementation. Warfarin remains the most commonly used anticoagulant in the United Kingdom. It is the third most common cause of adverse drug reactions leading to hospitalization, and approximately 40 percent of the variation in dose among patients is ascribed to two genes, *VKORC1* and *CYP2C9*, Turner said.

He summarized the main findings of the three pivotal, randomized controlled trials of genotype-guided warfarin dosing. The EU-PACT study found a statistically significant benefit with a genotyping strategy versus a standard loading strategy (Pirmohamed et al., 2013). The simultaneously published Clarification of Optimal Anticoagulation through Genetics (COAG) study, however, did not find genotype-guided dosing to have greater benefit than clinically guided dosing (Kimmel et al., 2013). The more recent GIFT trial, which Turner noted was powered for clinical endpoints, found the genotype strategy to have a statistically significant reduction in the primary clinical composite endpoint versus standard dosing (Gage et al., 2017). Together, the balance of evidence is in favor of warfarin pharmacogenomics, he said.

One potential reason why the COAG trial did not show a benefit was that there was more racial heterogeneity among the COAG trial participants, Turner postulated. More than 97 percent of the EU-PACT participants were Caucasian. In contrast, the COAG trial participants were 67 percent Caucasian, 27 percent African American, and 6 percent Hispanic. African American participants actually fared worse in the genotype arm compared to the clinical dosing algorithm, he said, which might be due to the fact that the COAG study did not take into account genotype variants that are specific to African Americans (Cavallari and Perera, 2012). This demonstrates the need to be mindful of evaluating genotypes that are pertinent to the specific patient population being treated, he said.

Another point to note is that the EU-PACT trial was carried out in Sweden and the United Kingdom, and genotyping was found to be likely more cost effective in the United Kingdom than in Sweden (Verhoef et al., 2016). It is plausible that this is due to Sweden being better at managing warfarin than the United Kindgom, in which case the incremental benefit of a pharmacogenomic strategy would probably be less in Sweden than in the United Kingdom, Turner suggested.

On this foundation, a small warfarin pharmacogenomics implementation initiative was launched in the northwest area of England. The initiative employed point-of-care testing to inform warfarin prescribing at three different hospitals. One of the sites was not as effective at recruiting participants as the other two sites, Turner said. Feedback from the research nurses indicated that the staff at that site felt they were too busy to take part in and learn the process. They felt that direct-acting oral anticoagulants were already better, and they did not seem to have much belief in pharmacogenomics, he said. This experience shows the need to become more inclusive and ensure that knowledge is being shared and education is being provided to practitioners up front to help overcome institutional cultural barriers.

100,000 Genomes Project

The last implementation initiative Turner described was the U.K.-wide 100,000 Genomes Project, which is conducting whole-genome sequencing of approximately 75,000 individuals to obtain 100,000 genomes: 75,000 germline genomes and 25,000 somatic genomes.[6] Participants are being recruited through 13 genomic medicine centers throughout the United Kingdom, which are hubs for a total of more than 80 different health care trusts. The genomic information is being entered into a data storage center and is being supplemented with clinical information from both the hospital and the primary care environment, when available. Researchers can access this information by joining Genomics England Clinical Interpretation Partnerships. Information is accessible through a virtual private network, but individual-level data cannot be downloaded. All activities are monitored, which, Turner said, ensures that access to the data is provided on an equitable basis, while assuring patients that their data are being appropriately handled.

---

[6]For more information on the 100,000 Genomes Project, see https://www.genomicsengland.co.uk/the-100000-genomes-project (accessed January 3, 2018).

Incentives to Collaborate and Share Data

One main incentive for collaboration and data sharing, Turner said, is funding, as was the case for the Ubiquitous Pharmacogenomics consortium. The ability to increase statistical power, enhance recruitment, and create economies of scale are other incentives for collaboration and data sharing. Working in collaboration can also offer risk mitigation and shared solutions (e.g., the ability to streamline ethical approvals by working together). Finally, as sample sizes increase, there is the potential for greater impact and greater ability to show clinical utility and cost effectiveness.

IDEAL MEASURES FOR GENOMIC MEDICINE IMPLEMENTATION STUDIES

Understanding implementation is critical for moving genomics from research into clinical care, Orlando said. Genomics researchers generally have a project and corresponding funding, and they figure out how make the project work, handling challenges as they come along. The downside of this approach, Orlando said, is that no one learns from these one-off solutions. Implementation without structure provides no guidance on implementation in other settings. The solutions are not generalizable and provide no model for the development of sustainability, she said.

Implementation scientists focus on creating generalizable approaches. As an example, Orlando mentioned the work of Peter Pronovost and colleagues on reducing central line infections. Applying an implementation science approach, they used a checklist-based intervention to significantly reduce infections. The key to success, Orlando explained, was not what was on the checklist, but the process of creating the checklist at each clinical site. Each institution tailored the intervention to its own site based on its issues and workflow.

Applying an implementation science approach could help advance the field of genomics, Orlando said. Clinical trials use traditional measures to assess the outcomes of various interventions. However, clinical trials exist within a larger framework, and elements of that framework affect how those trials are conducted and how effective they are. Those implementation elements (including clinician behavior) are not frequently measured. Standardized implementation measures are needed to assess implementation outcomes that in turn will affect traditional clinical utility outcomes, Orlando said.

The IGNITE Network

The Implementing Genomics in Practice (IGNITE) network is currently funding six different genomic intervention projects.[7] Each of the six research sites is implementing a different genomic intervention alongside a community partner. The goal is to create shared knowledge about the implementation experience and to facilitate knowledge transfer to others interested in implementing genomic interventions in their own health care settings.

The research sites in the IGNITE network have agreed to use an implementation science–based approach to their studies, and the Consolidated Framework for Implementation Research (CFIR) was used as the guiding framework for the network. The difference between a framework and a model, Orlando said, is that a framework essentially lists constructs, while a model describes relationships, such as how particular constructs inform an outcome. The CFIR compiled all of the existing models and data pertaining to implementation and presented them as a series of constructs. Overall there are 25 constructs and 13 sub-constructs, organized into five domains, outlined in Box 4-1 (Damschroder et al., 2009).

Using the CFIR constructs as a starting point, the IGNITE network's Common Measures Working Group identified constructs that were particularly important for genomic medicine, Orlando said. The resulting list was used to help develop new measures and create a common dataset across all of the projects. The list has been revisited several times as new sites and affiliates have become involved. The CFIR constructs and sub-constructs that ranked the highest for relevance to genomic medicine included costs, evidence strength and quality, available resources, leadership engagement, and champions, she said. Constructs that were ranked second highest included relative advantage, adaptability, complexity, patient needs and resources, implementation climate, relative priority, internal implementation leaders, planning, and executing. These are the aspects that people conducting implementation projects should consider measuring, Orlando said. Not all of the constructs have established measures. Although the Common Measures Working Group has developed several measures, additional measures are still needed, she said.

Because the characteristics of the patient are not currently part of the CFIR, a list of non-CFIR constructs was also developed. Non-CFIR patient measures identified thus far include demographics, self-reported health, health care activation, the social determinants of health, information sharing, health literacy, family and community assessments, attitude toward

---

[7]For more information on the IGNITE network, see https://ignite-genomics.org (accessed January 3, 2018).

BOX 4-1
CFIR Framework of Implementation
Constructs and Sub-Constructs

- **Intervention characteristics**—intervention source; evidence strength and quality; relative advantage; adaptability; trialability; complexity; design quality; cost.
- **Outer setting**—patient needs and resources; cosmopolitanism; peer pressure; external policies and incentives.
- **Inner setting**—structural characteristics; networks and communications; culture; implementation climate (*sub-constructs: tension for change; compatibility; relative priority; organizational incentives and rewards; goals and feedback; learning climate; leadership engagement; available resources; access to information and knowledge*).
- **Individuals involved**—knowledge and beliefs about the intervention; self-efficacy; individual stage of change; individual identification with the organization; other personal attributes.
- **Implementation process**—planning; engaging (*sub-constructs: opinion leaders; internal implementation leaders; champions, external change agents*); executing; reflecting and evaluating.

SOURCES: Lori Orlando, National Academies of Sciences, Engineering, and Medicine workshop presentation, November 1, 2017. Originally from Damschroder et al., 2009.

---

genomic intervention, and preference for who returns results. Additional patient measures will be added over time, Orlando said.

The working group also drafted and recently published a genomic medicine implementation research model, incorporating the constructs identified, how they interact, and how they might affect interventions (Orlando et al., 2017). Using an implementation science framework to guide genomic intervention implementations provides several additional benefits, Orlando said. First, it provides a broader frame for assessing health disparities. It also increases the reach of the intervention and allows for more generalizable interventions. Finally, it can increase the effectiveness of the intervention.

In summary, Orlando said that including system measures along with traditional measures and outcomes will help create sustainable interventions. The IGNITE network is a test bed for implementation research. A draft genomic medicine implementation research model is available, Orlando said, adding that her group is looking for opportunities to refine it. A method for identifying high-priority CFIR constructs has been developed

for others to use, and a list of non-CFIR high-priority constructs is in progress and should be updated with work that others are doing in this area.

DISCUSSION

The Role of EHRs

Several of the projects that were discussed earlier, such as eMERGE
and IGNITE, rely on EHRs, Grodman noted, and he asked panelists to
comment on the role of EHRs in the implementation of genomics-based
programs and, specifically, on whether the incorporation of the EHR is
necessary for implementation, or whether there are alternatives.

Association with the EHR is necessary, Chisholm said, and it is unlikely
that an alternative would be developed at this point. There will be opportunities to rethink how EHR systems are constructed (e.g., cloud based,
smartphone accessible, etc.) and how to improve the quality of the data
being captured (e.g., standards). The rate-limiting step, he said, is that
most people who enter data into EHRs have a very limited amount of time
for the patient encounter and EHR data entry. A key question for genomic
medicine implementation is how best to get the data out of the EHR,
Chisholm continued. He acknowledged that most genomics researchers do
not use the EHR, instead working with some sort of data extraction or data
mining approach that captures the EHR data and reconfigures it to be more
amenable to searching. An essential element for functionality is the ability
to use natural language processing and other approaches to capture data
that have been entered in the EHR as free text.

Another important aspect to consider is how best to enter genomic
test results into the EHR, Chisholm said. Clinical decision support has
been mentioned multiple times throughout the workshop, he noted. It is
important to monitor how often the pharmacogenomic decision support
tool is triggered and how often the physician overrides the recommendation (which, he added, is a significant percentage of the time). With regard
to genomic results, it is unlikely that whole-genome sequences would be
entered into the EHR, he said, as it would be an overwhelming amount of
data. There is some precedent for not entering medical data into the EHR,
he said. For example, medical imaging is not entered into the EHR, but
instead is accessible through a separate picture archiving and communication system (PACS). The eMERGE network has been considering ancillary
genomic systems (analogous to a PACS) and the rules that would be applied
to move information from the ancillary system to the EHR. As ClinVar and
ClinGen evolve, they might provide some of the rules that can be used to
move those data.

The EHR is a necessary part of modern health care, Boerwinkle said, but there are a lot of demands being placed on this relatively new technology, both in health care and in research. EHR tools are continuously evolving to become more useful, primarily for the quality of health care. There have been changes in the attitude of EHR vendors, who are now moving beyond the use of EHR for billing to using it to improve the quality of health care, Boerwinkle said, noting that the vendors seem much more engaged in trying to incorporate new information, including genomics.

Using the EHR on a daily basis is part of a clinician's job, and it represents a significant improvement compared to prior approaches to managing patient data, Orlando said. However, it can be burdensome for a clinician to have to enter the numerous diagnosis codes requested by researchers. Natural language processing, common data models, and data standards may help both clinicians and researchers improve data collection, Orlando said. Her research project for IGNITE has used SMART on FHIR (Substitutable Medical Applications, Reusable Technologies on Fast Healthcare Interoperability Resources) to integrate a family history tool into the EHR, helping both clinicians and researchers.

To ensure equity and inclusivity for patients and to engage as many clinicians as possible, involvement in genomic or pharmacogenomic implementation endeavors should be limited to hospitals that already have EHR systems, Turner said. Some necessary information is still not routinely collected (e.g., quality of life, drug adherence), which can be frustrating for researchers, he said. Natural language processing might help, but there is also a need to educate clinicians to collect this information.

Implementation Science in Practice

Less than 2 percent of the National Institutes of Health genomics research portfolio currently includes implementation science–based approaches (Roberts et al., 2017). Implementation science frameworks may represent an opportunity to design genomics-based screening programs in health care systems in such a way that proper data can be obtained that would indicate if the routine use of genomics in clinical practice is appropriate (NASEM, 2016).

Within the IGNITE network, there is currently only one implementation scientist, so there is an opportunity to bring in additional expertise in this space. There are also opportunities for bringing eMERGE and the Clinical Sequencing Evidence-Generating Research (CSER) consortium together to consider using the implementation science–based framework for the return of results and to address multiple other questions specific to genomics that an implementation science approach could help to answer, Orlando said.

The time may be right to bring implementation science tools and approaches to the return of results, Chisholm agreed. It will be important to conduct experiments to determine the appropriate way to proceed, rather than settling on a common framework up front, he said. Those involved with the All of Us research program plan to adopt a centralized model for storing data and providing access to those data. The data will be held at a central location, and the researchers will be brought to the data, rather than the data being taken to the researchers. This means that the data will be stored in a standardized format and common tools for analysis will be developed, Chisholm said. Still, there is space for experimentation and implementation science to better define approaches to querying data and returning results.

A traditional implementation science approach may not be working for genomic medicine, and it is not clear why, Boerwinkle said. There is a need to step back and ask why integrating genomics into routine health care is not happening, despite successful implementation science studies. One possible reason for the lack of widespread adoption is that there is not yet enough evidence accumulated on the clinical utility of such an integration. For a small part of the genome, such as variants found in the diseases designated as Tier 1 by the Centers for Disease Control and Prevention (e.g., hereditary breast and ovarian cancer, Lynch syndrome, and familial hypertension), it may be time for implementation. Within that implementation space, experimentation is important, Boerwinkle said, because it will be helpful to determine the best way to implement an evidence-based recommendation for cascade screening. Most pharmacogenomics, however, is in the Tier 2 space, where there is information about clinical validity but limited evidence about clinical utility.

Differences in Quality Among Genetic Testing Laboratories

There are more than 700 different laboratories across the United States doing genetic testing, and it is difficult to determine if the products coming out of these laboratories are equivalent in quality, said a workshop participant. When data are not shared, there is a risk of the testing being duplicated—for example, when a patient changes insurers. This can be wasteful, assuming that the quality of the product from different laboratories is the same, the participant added.

Like any clinical laboratory, there is a range of quality for genetic testing laboratories, Chisholm said. Data sharing may actually feed back into the system and improve quality over time. ClinGen has conducted analyses of different laboratories, including analyses of their annotation processes and the curation of the variants that they have labeled as pathogenic, likely pathogenic, or benign. Where discrepancies were found, ClinGen helped to adjudicate those discrepancies, and build tools to help resolve them, Chisholm noted. Some of the discrepancies were simply due to addition errors in the score used to determine whether a variant is pathogenic or likely pathogenic. Some individuals have suggested that payers should cover testing only for those who are willing to have their data entered into ClinVar, so that it can be evaluated, Chisholm said, which would have huge impact on data quality from the laboratories.

In his experience as founder of a genetic testing laboratory and as a former chair of the American Clinical Lab Association, Grodman said, most clinical laboratories operate under the strict standards of the Clinical Laboratory Improvement Amendments and the College of American Pathologists, as well as stringent state requirements. Genetic testing takes place in both academic centers and clinical reference laboratories, and in both cases the goal is to provide a quality result. However, it is important to be aware that the knowledge about the pathogenicity of variants can change in the future, and that does not mean that a laboratory did the test wrong or that it did not work, Grodman said.

Data Sharing Incentives for the Long Term

NHGRI has funded innovative research programs such as eMERGE, CSER, and IGNITE, which facilitate information sharing among researchers and health care systems. It is important to identify the incentives for health care systems to participate in massive data sharing networks and to share data across systems, in the event that the research programs are no longer supported by government funding, Ginsburg said. Some forward-thinking health care systems are building capability, which clearly advances their own research agenda and perhaps their clinical agenda (to be competitive in their local environments), he said, but what happens to data sharing when IGNITE, CSER, and eMERGE cease to exist?

Demonstrating the value of data sharing is important, Chisholm said. For example, the Chicago Area Patient-Centered Outcomes Research Network is a clinical data research network that shares the movement of participants among different health care systems in the Chicago area (discussed by Kho in Chapter 5). There is value in understanding how porous a health care system is and how frequently people are moving between health care systems, he said. From both quality-of-care and cost-management perspectives, there is value in knowing that a patient who frequently presents at one emergency department is also presenting in emergency departments elsewhere in the area.

At the most basic level, institutions will be driven to promote data sharing when sharing becomes an integral part of quality, management, and reimbursement metrics, Boerwinkle said. Data from the HealthConnect experience show that the number of frequent users of health services is much higher than previously thought. Frequent users were previously defined as those who were repeatedly using the same health care system. When systems are connected, it becomes clear that people are moving around among them. Patients are going to demand data sharing and really drive it through programs such as Sync for Science,[8] Boerwinkle said. Because the funding situation is different in the United Kingdom, Turner said, data sharing is being driven by the pursuit of clinical utility and cost effectiveness. Evidence of cost effectiveness (not just in the United Kingdom, but worldwide) would drive governments to support it, because it would save money for the system overall.

Data Sharing by Individuals

The concept of allowing individuals to share their data as a potential solution was revisited by a workshop participant. Although there are advantages to this mechanism, there are also many practical barriers. For example, the infrastructure, data tools, and money are given to institutions that have intellectual property rights and goals for their programs. There are privacy and security concerns that are significant and costly. How could individual data sharing be implemented practically? The barriers are not insurmountable if individuals are empowered, Boerwinkle said, and they could be empowered by a clear policy decision such as a court decision that dictates that individuals have authority over their own data. The barriers will begin to wither after the first steps are taken. A first step of creating a data marketplace, or some incentive for people to focus on individual data sharing, could move this concept forward. The Genetic Alliance is one organization trying to do this, according to a workshop participant, but there are practical and infrastructure challenges. It is not useful if individuals have access to their data but have nowhere to share the data or no easy mechanism to do so.

---

[8]Sync for Science is a collaboration among researchers, EHR vendors, and the U.S. federal government. For more information on the project, see http://syncfor.science (accessed January 18, 2018).

5

Understanding Participant Needs and Preferences and Improving Diversity and Equity

---

Highlights of Key Points Made by Individual Speakers

- Policies developed with public participation are more likely to be perceived as legitimate and trusted and therefore have a better chance at successful implementation. A multi-way, iterative dialogue among researchers and participants about what people may or may not want to learn from whole-genome sequencing is needed. (Knight)

- Assumptions are often made that concerns expressed by certain groups are race based; however, that is not necessarily the case. When designing community-based care and health care systems, consider diversity broadly to be inclusive of race, ethnicity, education, culture, socioeconomic status, and access to resources. (Knight)

- Look to other disciplines to learn from their successes in creating a more diverse research workforce and research programs that engage diverse populations. (Horowitz)

- There are significant financial incentives for quality improvement within health care systems. If research goals can be aligned with quality improvement initiatives, a sizable amount of funding can be used to support the research infrastructure. (Kho)

> • Engaging diverse populations where they are (i.e., being sensitive to context) and involving them in the decision-making process is valuable and necessary to ensuring equity when designing genomics-based programs. (Horowitz, Kho, Knight)

In this session, panelists considered the policy issues associated with the implementation of genomics-based programs in health care systems and potentially in public health. Topics discussed included approaches to ensuring data security and participant privacy and methods for supporting equity and accessibility in genomics-based programs. Sara Knight, a professor in the Division of Preventive Medicine at the University of Alabama at Birmingham, discussed her work on understanding participant needs and addressing issues of diversity and equity in genomic health services. Carol Horowitz, a professor of population health science and policy at Mount Sinai Hospital in New York City, described the collection of genetic data from a diverse population while keeping the perspectives of the community in mind. Abel Kho, the director of the Center for Health Information Partnerships at Northwestern University, described the work of Pastors4PCOR as an example of taking research out into the community. The session was moderated by Vence Bonham, a senior advisor to the Director on Genomics and Health Disparities at NHGRI.

PARTICIPANT NEEDS, DIVERSITY, AND EQUITY[1]

One of the important elements to consider when developing services is what patients need and want, Knight said. She described a series of studies designed to better understand patient preferences related to genomic testing, including a study examining preferences for Lynch syndrome screening in the general population and studies about integrating genomic screening in the Department of Veterans Affairs (VA). In all of these efforts, Knight emphasized the importance of shared decision making for ensuring diversity and equity in programs.

Patient, Public, and Clinician Preferences

The first study that Knight described was designed to understand preferences for genetic testing for Lynch syndrome (Walsh et al., 2012). Inter-

---

[1]Knight clarified that the views expressed in her presentation are her own views, and do not necessarily reflect the position or the policy of the Department of Veterans Affairs, the National Cancer Institute, the National Human Genome Research Institute, or the U.S. government.

views and focus groups were conducted with patients at high risk for Lynch syndrome and with members of the public who were interested in Lynch syndrome screening. The participants were very enthusiastic overall, Knight said. Responses indicated that those who participated in the focus groups were willing to pay for the test, that they were very concerned about false negative results (i.e., actually having a condition that was not picked up in a screening test), and that they associated genetic testing with health benefits. Clinicians were also surveyed, and their concerns focused on guidelines for screening and the patient and family psychosocial experience (e.g., anxiety), including potential downstream harms.

The results of the first study on preferences for genetic testing for Lynch syndrome were used to design a Web-based survey, including a discrete choice experiment, to understand the characteristics of genetic testing that might influence preferences for getting tested. A probability-based online group of 355 U.S. residents aged 50 and over was surveyed in April 2010 (Knight et al., 2015). Knight noted that these were individuals who would most likely already have had experience with colorectal cancer screening because U.S. Preventive Services Task Force guidelines recommend routine screening starting at age 50. In response to the "best" test scenario, in which the test results would be shared with the primary care provider and there was a zero percent chance of false negative results, the researchers found that 97 percent of those surveyed would opt for using genetic testing. In the "worst" test scenario, test results would be shared with life and health insurance companies and there was a 20 percent false negative rate. In this case, 41 percent would choose to use genetic testing, although as Knight added, the survey was conducted around the same time that the Patient Protection and Affordable Care Act (ACA) was enacted, and this may have changed some perceptions surrounding preexisting conditions and insurability. The results demonstrated that the interest in and use of genomic services varies depending on participant preferences and also on the setting and conditions that surround the test, Knight said.

Incorporating Genomics into Routine Care for Veterans

Knight continued this line of study within the VA, conducting a retrospective cohort analysis of how genomics was being incorporated into routine care for veterans with colon cancer. This was followed by key informant interviews with clinicians in the Veterans Health Administration (VHA) to identify the barriers to and facilitators of routine genomic services for colorectal cancer patients.

The sample cohort included all veterans under age 50 in the VHA system who had been diagnosed with colorectal cancer between 2003 and 2010. The majority were men, which is typical for samples collected from the VHA, Knight noted. Thirty-five percent were African American. Many of the individuals in the cohort had been diagnosed with late-stage tumors (stages 3 and 4). Knight said that the average age was 46 (with a range of 19 to 55 years), indicating that many of these individuals may not have been diagnosed through screening. At the time of the study (2003–2010), many of the guidelines recommended that those under age 50 diagnosed with colorectal cancer be given immunohistochemistry (IHC) and microsatellite instability (MSI) testing of tumor tissue to determine whether genetic testing for Lynch syndrome would be recommended. This molecular analysis of tumor tissue is a relatively low-cost approach for decision making about genetic testing, Knight noted. She shared unpublished data that indicated a marked increase in use of IHC and MSI testing in the VA beginning in 2010 as the systematic implementation of molecular analysis of tumor tissue was initiated, and she said that another cohort that captures the full implementation effort is now being assessed.

In a study of barriers to and facilitators of genomic health services in the VA, Knight and colleagues interviewed VA clinicians and administrators about their experiences referring veterans diagnosed with colorectal cancer for genetic counseling, molecular analysis of tumor tissue, and genetic testing. Clinicians from both high-oncology-volume facilities and low-oncology-volume facilities were interviewed, including oncologists, gastroenterologists, and primary care physicians (Sperber et al., 2016). Molecular testing of tumors was seen as low-cost and advantageous for decision making, Knight said, though most clinicians responded that they saw few cases of younger patients diagnosed with colorectal cancer and infrequently used molecular tumor tissue testing. Clinicians also noted that there were no request and approval routines in place in the VHA at that time. Clinicians were interested in the opportunity to consult with experts, such as clinical geneticists or genetic counselors, but they said that there was no standard referral process and that some referrals went through gatekeepers, which made the process time consuming. Clinicians (including oncologists and gastroenterologists) thought that they did not have the expertise to talk with patients about genetics and genomics. They perceived that information on genetics and genomics would be valuable for their patients, but they did not know where to obtain the expertise within the VHA. These findings on the lack of expertise in genetics and genomics suggest an opportunity for education, Knight said, given the limited workforce in genetic counseling and clinical genetics in VA and non-VA health care settings.

Aligning Genomic Health Services with the Values and Preferences of Veterans from Diverse Backgrounds

A study now under way at the VA is aimed at informing the design of a genomic medicine service in the VHA that would be aligned with the preferences and needs of veterans from diverse backgrounds.[2] The study seeks to understand veterans' preferences for the return of results from whole-genome sequencing. Knight briefly described some of the challenges that can be encountered when trying to understand population perspectives on genomics using methods such as advisory committees, focus groups, surveys of convenience samples, and consensus panels. Each of these methods alone is limited in its ability to provide a generalizable picture of the types of genomic health care services that would be valued in diverse populations.

To address these challenges, Knight and her colleagues are using a mixed methods design beginning with interviews and focus groups of 120 veterans from four geographic regions of the United States (Northeast, Southeast, South Central, and Western) to assess the types of results that veterans would find valuable from whole-genome sequencing and the types of health care services they would want in order to understand and use the results. The focus group data will be used to construct a discrete choice experiment survey that will be tested for relevance to the VA and then delivered to a large random sample of veterans drawn from all veterans cared for in the VHA. Minority veterans will be oversampled, and the overall sample will be of sufficient sample size to examine differences in values and preferences across subgroups of veterans. The random sample of veterans from diverse sociodemographic groups will provide generalizable information on veterans' preferences for the return of results from whole-genome sequencing.

The study was designed to comprehensively engage veterans and key VHA health care system leaders with researchers in the dissemination of findings in the VHA. Using a democratic deliberation method, VA stakeholders, including clinicians, policy makers, and veterans, will be educated about the integrated results of the focus groups, interviews, and survey and given an opportunity for informed discussion as a group to ultimately help define priorities for veteran-centered genomic testing and to inform VA efforts to develop policies for the return of results from whole-genome sequencing.

---

[2] For more information, see https://www.hsrd.research.va.gov/research/abstracts.cfm?Project_ID=2141705720 (accessed January 24, 2018).

Multi-Level, Multi-Process Stakeholder Engagement

In conclusion, Knight emphasized the need for a multi-way, iterative dialogue among veterans affected by policies on genomic health care services, health services researchers, and policy makers. She said that policies developed with public participation are more likely to be perceived as legitimate and trusted and are more likely to be implemented. Her studies are now using a highly nuanced, multi-level, multi-process stakeholder engagement process that involves in-depth key informant interviews and representative surveys to inform ethical considerations, research methods, and translational activities; advisory boards of patients, family members, clinicians, health system leaders, and community leaders; and democratic deliberative process groups to engage the public, policy makers, and clinicians in the development of sensible genomic health care policies and genomic medicine programs that can be implemented in diverse communities and health care systems.

ENGAGING DIVERSE POPULATIONS IN GENOMICS-BASED RESEARCH

Horowitz began by sharing some perspectives from her diverse partners on a genomics stakeholder board (Kaplan et al., 2017). The board was formed to help guide the genomics work of the Center for Health Equity and Community Engaged Research at the Icahn School of Medicine at Mount Sinai in New York City and is composed of patients, advocates, clinicians, researchers, systems leaders, funders, and industry representatives. Horowitz listed a series of questions the board members have considered as they move forward with research in their community:

- **Whose decision is it to integrate genomics?** In other words, who needs to agree that genomic testing can bring value (e.g., payers, providers, patients, policy makers, researchers)? Understanding the audience for the evidence will determine the kinds of research questions that need to be asked.
- **Who is at the table nationally and locally?** Who is participating in the discussions and making decisions regarding what questions need to be asked, how those questions will be answered, and what will be done with the results?
- **If genomics is not studied, will it happen anyway?** If we do not study genomics, the board asked, who will, and in which patients? The answer to that question often comes down to funding. If only academic medical centers are funded to do genomics research, then it will only be patients who go to academic medical centers

who are part of the research. It is important to reach out to more diverse sites, Horowitz said. The conclusion of the board was, she said, "One needs to be vigilant. The research should proceed, but carefully."

- **Can genomics-based research reach diverse participants and be equitably distributed?** The answer is yes, Horowitz said, if the research is intentional, valued, resourced, and done carefully. She shared the input of one community partner who asked how science can be advanced in a good way, while not taking advantage of the vulnerability of a community. Horowitz observed that stereotypes and paternalistic attitudes can promote concerns among researchers about engaging minority populations that are unfounded, and she recalled one community partner who suggested that genomics can be integrated into community health in an equitable way. It is important to recognize who is rejecting whom, Horowitz said. Are communities really saying they do not have an interest in genomics, she asked, or are providers and researchers focusing on implementing where they have already been successful because it may be less difficult?

APOL1 Risk Variants

As an example of the collection of genetic data from a diverse population with the perspectives of the community in mind, Horowitz described the Genetic Testing to Understand and Address Renal Disease Disparities (GUARDD) study,[3] a study examining the risk variants of the apolipoprotein L1 gene (*APOL1*).

People of African ancestry have a risk of kidney failure that is about three to four times higher than people of Caucasian or European ancestry (NIDDK, 2016). One out of seven people of African ancestry carries a genetic variant of *APOL1* that increases the odds of kidney failure approximately tenfold if the individual has hypertension, Horowitz said (Genovese et al., 2010; Horowitz et al., 2017). This finding can explain up to 70 percent of the racial disparity in kidney failure, she said. Horowitz noted that she first became aware of this disparity when it was raised at a community board meeting. As a researcher, she felt it was necessary to have patient and community support to pursue any research in this area. After approaching a genetic ethicist for advice, Horowitz was initially advised against any race- or ancestry-based genomics research, being told that it would "set the disparities movement back 30 years." However, when Horowitz spoke

---

[3]For more information on the GUARDD study, see https://ignite-genomics.org/sites/mount-sinai (accessed January 12, 2018).

with community leader Mimsie Robinson of the Bethel Gospel Assembly in New York, he was in favor of pursuing this research topic because gaining a better understanding of common genetic variants in African Americans associated with kidney disease might help to alleviate possible providers' stereotypes that black patients are sick due to non-compliance or other negative attitudes or behaviors (Horowitz et al., 2017).

The GUARDD study is a randomized controlled trial funded by NHGRI as part of the IGNITE network. The study enrolled adults of self-reported African ancestry with hypertension and without diabetes or kidney disease, Horowitz said. Participants were randomized to *APOL1* testing immediately, or delayed testing 1 year later. Because the availability of genetic counselors was limited, it was decided, with input from participants and providers, that local community residents with college degrees would be trained by genetic counselors to return results to participants with oversight from the counselors.

A community–clinical–academic team developed the study methodology. The process began with formative research, introducing GUARDD at five federally qualified health centers, six neighborhood practices, and four academic primary care practices throughout New York City. At each site, the proposal was presented to the providers for their feedback. Many of the providers did not have much experience with genomics or research, Horowitz said. The recruitment strategy was developed by the team with the participants in mind, and Horowitz called it "a good invitation to a good party." In other words, consider who the target audience is, and be flexible with when and where those people can participate. Recruiters were drawn from the community, and recruitment materials were developed with appropriate graphics and language and at appropriate literacy levels.

Enrollment of over 2,000 participants was completed in 2 years. At 3 months, 93 percent of participants were retained, and at 12 months, 88 percent. Horowitz noted that this was a difficult-to-reach population with some people experiencing extreme social stressors such as homelessness and recent incarceration and others having competing demands with jobs and professional conflicts. Despite this, there was a very low refusal rate (only 12 percent of eligible participants refused to join the study). All participants were of African ancestry, but they were diverse in other ways: 20 percent had low health literacy, 44 percent had less than a high school diploma, 53 percent had income under $30,000, 48 percent were non-adherent to their blood pressure medications, and 47 percent had uncontrolled blood pressure.

Based on a survey of the providers recruited to the study, about half were non-white. Of those, half were Asian, and half were black or Latino. Most of these clinicians responded that they had taken a formal genetics course, but only one-third had ordered a genetic test for a patient in the last year. Even fewer (one-fourth) felt prepared to communicate results with patients who had genetic tests for chronic diseases. More than half of the providers responded that they had concerns about insurance discrimination, and more than three-quarters said they did not trust genetic testing companies. Most providers indicated that race and ancestry were good clues as to who should undergo genetic testing and that genes may play a role in existing health disparities.

A baseline survey of the beliefs and concerns of the 2,000 study participants revealed that few had ever had a previous genetic test or understood genetic testing. Despite that, Horowitz said, nearly all thought it was a good idea to get genetic testing to assess chronic disease risk. Most also wanted their children to be tested for *APOL1* variants. Preliminary results 3 months later, after tests had been done and results had been returned, found that nearly all would get tested again and were satisfied with the timing, type, and amount of information they received.

Preliminary clinical results of the study suggest that participants who were told they had high-risk genetic variants had a greater decrease in systolic blood pressure at 3 months, Horowitz said, which was associated with self-reported improvements in blood pressure medication use. More detailed results from the study are expected to be published later in 2018.

Exploring Lessons Learned

In conclusion, Horowitz said, diverse populations and sites should not be just a funding strategy for studies. Patients and community partners emphasized that if researchers want to learn about them, then they need to be included. Partners also said that "the culture of understanding is far more important than the culture of fear, and the culture of understanding has no color." Finally, patients and community partners need to have their voices harnessed, Horowitz said, adding that "people become engaged when someone who looks like them is at the helm." She concluded her presentation with a message from her community partners: "Do the research now, do it right, and make diversity and engagement a priority from the get-go. Don't make it an afterthought."

CLOSING THE CIRCLE BETWEEN RESEARCH AND THE COMMUNITY

There are very good scientific reasons for having diversity in research, Kho said. He referred participants to the work of Green and colleagues on the ecology of care as an example (Green et al., 2001). Using administrative data, Green and his colleagues described how people use the health care system and followed the health care journeys of people who came in to see a provider over the course of a month. In 1 month, for every 1,000 people, 800 reported symptoms of illness, 217 visited a physician's office, fewer received care in other health venues (complementary or alternative care provider, hospital outpatient clinic, home health care, emergency department), 8 were hospitalized, and 1 or fewer were hospitalized in an academic medical center. Most research is conducted in academic medical centers, Kho noted. Overall, during the 1-month study period, only about 22 percent of the people in the study had seen any provider at all. This finding indicates that population studies, including genomics-based screening programs, may miss about 80 percent of the targeted group, which highlights the need for research to go out into the community, Kho said.

Kho described a similar analysis performed by his group using recent data to estimate how many people actually have their data captured in an electronic health record (EHR) in a given month. His analysis suggests that 20 percent of individuals studied are seen by a provider in a given month and therefore have a chance of having their data captured in the EHR. An additional challenge with EHR data is that they are fragmented across institutions. On average, about 20 percent of any person's information is likely missing across systems, Kho continued. If a patient goes to one health system, there is a good chance that there is some record of that person in another system within the network (Kho et al., 2015). The extent varies somewhat across different conditions. For a patient with type 2 diabetes, for example, looking at one institution provides only a portion of that person's record. Looking across all of the systems in that area gathers about 20 percent more data. Furthermore, only about one in five people in a community will have EHR data of any quality. From a genomics standpoint, if research is tethered to EHR data, then phenotypic information for a vast proportion of the population will be missing in a pure, care-based approach. This is a potentially significant limitation, Kho said. While the EHR is a good resource if it is available, from an epidemiological standpoint, there are many places where there will not be EHR data. The question is how to obtain that wider set of information.

Kho said that his work has been focused on how to get out of the academic center and into the community. About half of his work focuses on quality improvement and measurement. He pointed out that there are significant financial incentives for quality improvement within the health care systems. If research goals can be aligned with the quality improvement initiatives of health care systems, a sizable amount of funding can be tapped to underwrite the research infrastructure, he said.

Pastors4PCOR

As an example of taking the research out into the community, Kho described the work of Pastors4PCOR, a Patient-Centered Outcomes Research Institute (PCORI)-funded community health outreach initiative engaging faith-based communities in Chicago's south side and south suburbs.[4] Kho suggested that Pastors4PCOR is actually the community engaging academia rather than the other way around. In this emerging model, when academia fails to sufficiently engage with the community, the community takes the initiative and engages researchers on its own terms. A group of community advocates and faith-based partners, including leaders from local churches, researchers from academic medical centers, and community health partners, came together to identify research priorities based on community interest.

Pastors4PCOR brings together these stakeholders to create a survey skills training program that allows community members to support the health and well-being of their communities. Essentially, Kho said, pastors and key members of the parishes are being trained to engage in research. The initiative is very effective at promoting research by focusing on being informed, having respect for the lived experience, trust, understanding the context of where community members are, and working together on issues that matter to all partners, he added. Over the past 2 years, Pastors4PCOR has been conducting health research ambassador workshops around Chicago and is now beginning to spread the movement to other areas in the United States, including Los Angeles and parts of Arkansas.

One of the most valuable lessons Kho said he has learned from Pastors4PCOR is to find an elegant way of distilling messages into something simple and understandable. For example, informed consent is explained as "making sure everyone knows what the study is about and understanding they can withdraw at any time," and confidentiality "requires a clear explanation of how data sharing will be respected and processed." "Voluntariness" is a term they use to describe how there should not be consequences for saying "no" to engaging in research. For example, participants should not be pressured, made to feel bad, threatened (e.g., with loss of services), or offered lots of money to take risks.

Surveys of the ambassadors-in-training show that they tend to be around age 50, with the majority (80 percent) female, and they are generally very well educated (75 percent have college degrees or higher). Although technology use in the wider population in Chicago is quite high, Kho said, the surveys show that while the ambassadors do use the Internet,

---

[4]For more information on Pastors4PCOR, see https://www.pcori.org/research-results/2015/pastors-4-pcor-engaging-faith-based-communities (accessed January 3, 2018).

smartphones, and e-mail, they do not use social media as much, which is becoming a bit of a challenge as they begin to engage in the research. The ambassadors ranked high blood pressure, diabetes, cancer, substance use issues, and mental health issues as the most prevalent health conditions in their faith-based communities, followed by obesity and gun violence. Kho noted that this was confirmed by looking at the co-localized distribution of the participating churches and the distribution of cases of hypertension and diabetes in Chicago. When the ambassadors were asked what they would like to learn more about from researchers, the top-ranked responses were cancer, high blood pressure, diabetes, mental health disorders, heart disease, and stroke. The top health-related factors that faith-based communities should focus on were identified as behavioral information and education, followed by support for mental health, access to health care, family and social support, access to healthy foods, and community safety. At the end of the 12-week training program, nearly all of the participants felt confident that they could communicate the concepts of patient-centered outcomes research back to the community in a way that would be effective.

To conclude, Kho briefly highlighted the PCORI-funded ADAPTABLE (Aspirin Dosing: A Patient-Centric Trial Assessing Benefits and Long-Term Effectiveness) trial as an example of one of the Pastors4PCOR projects. As discussed, hypertension, diabetes, and cardiovascular disease are priorities in many of the communities. Kho and colleagues are helping Pastors4PCOR drive the trial, though he noted that there have been quite a few unanticipated challenges. For example, there is very little in the way of infrastructure, including computer support. At the request of those involved with Pastors4PCOR, Northwestern has helped set them up with tablets and computers, which gives them the ability to check participant eligibility across the different systems in an anonymous way and to start recruitment.

DISCUSSION

To start the discussion, Bonham prompted panelists to suggest to the Roundtable one specific activity or focus area for increasing diversity in genomics-based programs. Knight recommended that the Roundtable carefully consider the types of diversity that are important to include when designing community-based care and health care systems (e.g., race, ethnicity, education, socioeconomic status, material hardship). Assumptions are often made that the fears or concerns expressed by certain groups are race based; however, that is not necessarily the case. Kho emphasized the need to get out into the community more often in order to bring in diverse perspectives. There is a lot of ongoing work that, while not focused on genomics, could potentially feed into genomics-based efforts. Horowitz suggested that the Roundtable could become more diverse or could form a "network of networks" to reach out to more diverse places for more diverse perspectives. Learning from other disciplines about their successes in creating a more diverse research workforce and research programs that engage diverse populations could also be helpful, Horowitz said. Genomics is a newcomer to translational research relative to some other disciplines, and it can learn from them, she added.

Participants considered ancestral versus genetic identity, genetic discrimination, and the equitable distribution of the benefits of genomics. Throughout the discussion, speakers highlighted the need to consider the context of implementation and to engage participants in a thoughtful way.

Genomics and Ancestral Identity

Horowitz said that participants were recruited to her study in real time based on their self-reports of having African ancestry (not being African American), as opposed to being genetically defined. This is an important distinction, she said, as the study was more about ancestry in genomics than race in genomics. In this case, there happened to be a close correlation between people who self-reported African ancestry and those who had genetic African ancestry, but determining genetic ancestry was not part of the study. Horowitz noted that the researchers spent considerable time consulting with a diverse group of experts and stakeholders to determine how best to ask community members about their African ancestry. The study also considered other social determinants of health and how they intersect with genomics, including depression, anxiety, racism, life chaos, food insufficiency, and other elements. Knight said that some of her studies ask very detailed questions about race, ethnicity, and ancestry, in part to attempt to recruit participants from groups underrepresented in genomics research, such as those of Asian and Indian ancestry.

When asked if researchers had concerns about not genetically confirming self-reported ancestry, which could potentially affect conclusions made from research, Horowitz emphasized the need for care and sensitivity in reporting genetic ancestry to individuals, and she noted the potential challenges of having to report to individuals that they do or do not actually have genetic evidence of the ancestry they identify with. Horowitz and Kho both noted their doubts about the usefulness of genetic confirmation of ancestry. It might be interesting from a methods standpoint, Kho said, but he agreed that handling discrepancies would be a challenge. Bonham said that his work is focused on better understanding social and cultural contexts and added his caution that in considering variation in the genome in relation to ancestral backgrounds, genomic measurement of identity is something that requires further discussion. Genomic information and variations across ancestral backgrounds hold promise for research, but contextual issues should be carefully considered, Horowitz and Bonham suggested, adding that the issues might be a topic for future discussion by the Roundtable.

Genetic Discrimination

Differences in policy may affect populations differently, said a workshop participant. For example, genomic screening studies or cascade testing of current or former members of the military could affect their careers or retention of benefits. Knight responded that veterans, military service members, and members of the federal government are not covered by the Genetic Information Nondiscrimination Act of 2008 (GINA); however, in her own research she has observed that veterans are covered by other policies that may actually be more protective of their rights than GINA. Understanding the Department of Defense and VA policies is important when reassuring people about their level of protection, so that a veteran or a military service member can make an informed decision about participating in genomic studies. Ethically, it is important to be aware of and thoughtful about the fact that the policies that govern their protections are different from the policies that govern the protection of most of the rest of the population.

Another participant asked whether the panelists had heard any concerns from communities about the potential for genetic discrimination and what can or should be done to ease those concerns, especially in light of anticipated changes to the ACA. As a provider, Kho voiced concern and added that health care systems appear to be concerned, and he said that he had observed distrust in communities. Knight said that the issues of privacy and protecting one's ability to get health care were identified as very important in her first preferences study. Her current study, which is a much larger, population-based study, will allow her to analyze subgroups (including veterans who are underserved and underinsured) for differences in their preferences and perspectives regarding data protections and participation. She said that in her first study there was optimism in the focus groups that the ACA would address concerns regarding preexisting conditions. There is greater concern now, however, and that concern will need to be taken into account as an important contextual variable in the current study. She said that she expects that the population-based survey would include questions to understand how the heightened concern about genetic discrimination might influence preferences and value.

Equitable Distribution of the Benefits of Genomics

Several individual participants highlighted several areas to consider when discussing diversity and equity in genomics-based programs, including disparities in access to and use of health care, rare diseases, health literacy, individuals with limited capacity to consent, and the use of trusted brokers to reach out to underserved populations.

One disparity to keep in mind is whether and how people are covered by health care benefits and the extent to which they use services, George Isham said. Uptake is variable, he noted, and is affected by social and other factors. When considering how health care systems can scale their approach to genomics in terms of databases and investment in large infrastructures to support programs, it is also important to consider how implementation can be done to ensure that the benefits of genomics are distributed more equitably across the population. In this regard, Kho highlighted the issue of data sharing by health care systems (see Chapter 4 for more information). He observed that there are commercial endeavors working toward collecting and linking all of the different types of data available for an individual, independent of the health care systems. Leaders of health care systems need to be thinking much more broadly about how to bring together the many elements of the health data world, where bits of data are strewn everywhere, he said.

The low prevalence of certain diseases is a challenge for genetic screening, said a workshop participant. Low-prevalence diseases include both rare diseases and diseases that are very specific to certain populations. The participant asked whether there are efforts to ensure that particular genetic screening tests are accessible to those groups that might be affected more than others and also asked about efforts to include data on rare diseases in databases. While highly prevalent conditions can be studied using population-based approaches, rare diseases are often brought to the forefront by the self-organization of those affected, Kho said. In many cases, families affected by rare diseases have pulled together to form registries, which are often quite deep and include informed consent models and biospecimens. Kho also noted that some of these groups have come forward asking to build a link to their disease in the EHR in order to advance research. He agreed that there is a need to find equitable approaches to using genomics to study rare diseases, and he emphasized that data have value and that it is important to ensure that the people whose data are being shared and used are reaping the benefits. Knight emphasized the importance of transparency when designing genomic medicine programs, adding that understanding the perspectives of different groups, some whom could benefit more and others who might benefit less, is critical to equitable system design and decision making.

Patients who have limited capacity to consent to research projects due to learning difficulties, delirium, dementia, or related conditions represent another area of diversity for consideration. These groups of patients are often underrepresented in studies, Turner said. Based on his experience, patients at the sickest end of the spectrum have comorbidities and polypharmacy that can be barriers to enrollment in studies; however, these patients could benefit from pharmacogenomics knowledge. Turner asked about any initiatives to include this cohort in genomics programs while also protecting and preserving their dignity. The field needs to think very broadly about the groups that are underrepresented in genomics research, Knight said. Another underserved population is people with multiple morbidities who live in highly rural areas in the southern United States, she added. Horowitz observed that some individuals who are thought to be unable to consent actually can consent when appropriate language, literacy level, and techniques are used (e.g., the teach back method). On the other hand, she cautioned, it is important not to coerce people or to assume understanding based on physical cues. Bonham added that the All of Us initiative is being very thoughtful about how it defines diversity and is considering factors beyond those of economics, race, and ethnicity.

Building trust with diverse groups to encourage participation in genomics is important, and having trusted brokers to facilitate communication and engagement with underserved or diverse populations would be helpful, said a workshop participant. The community health worker model has been found to be a very well-accepted way of engaging the community, Kho said, but there has to be a willingness to learn and listen based on the context of where you are. Horowitz suggested directly asking the group that you wish to engage with whom they trust. For example, some of the younger people in the communities they serve have become less trusting of churches, meaning that other trusted brokers need to be identified, she added. Asking small business owners and leaders in the business community in small southern towns to become more involved in stakeholder groups could be another solution, Knight said, because businesses are often a hub where people congregate. Business owners are very knowledgeable about their communities and can be influential as representatives of their communities on advisory boards or panels that are involved in engagement.

6

Improving Health Through the Integration of Genomics-Based Programs: Potential Next Steps

In the final session of the workshop, an emerging model for accelerating evidence generation for genomic technologies in a learning health care system was discussed. Several of the workshop panelists considered the benefits, costs, and harms of such models and addressed the policies and infrastructure needed to enable the sharing of genomic data across institutions. Individual speakers shared their thoughts on actionable next steps that could support the implementation of genomics-based programs in health care systems, and co-chairs Feero and Veenstra captured and summarized key themes that were discussed during the day on topics including evidence generation, data sharing, and genomics-based program design.

A MODEL FOR ACCELERATING EVIDENCE
GENERATION FOR GENOMIC TECHNOLOGIES
IN A LEARNING HEALTH CARE SYSTEM

There is limited evidence available on the clinical utility of most genomic tests (Phillips et al., 2017). To date, there have been very few randomized controlled trials looking at the clinical utility of genomic technologies, said Christine Lu, an associate professor in the Department of Population Medicine at Harvard Medical School. Randomized controlled trials are costly and lengthy and are often not suitable for the study of precision medicine. To address this problem, Lu described a proposed model for generating evidence of clinical utility. The model includes the assumption that the genetic tests under assessment for utility have proven analytical and clinical validity, she said. Although the model is designed to generate clinical utility evidence, Lu said, some of the data generated by the model could also be relevant for demonstrating economic utility. The model is focused on the Tier 2 genomic applications in the classification system devised by the Centers for Disease Control and Prevention (Dotson et al., 2014). Tier 1 applications, Lu explained, already have sufficient evidence of clinical utility to support adoption in clinical practice. By contrast, for Tier 2 applications there is early evidence of potential utility, but the evidence is not sufficient. Embedded in the model is the concept of a learning health care system, in which new data will inform continuous improvement of clinical practice and the larger health care system (Chambers et al., 2016; IOM, 2013, 2015).

Building Blocks for Rapid Evidence Generation

The model for rapid generation of evidence of clinical utility is based on three building blocks: temporary coverage, leveraging data networks, and stakeholder engagement and endorsement (Lu et al., 2017). Temporary coverage encourages the use of genomic tests. Temporary coverage is enabled by risk-sharing agreements and value-based contracts between manufacturers and payers. Clinical genomic test orders and results are captured by claims and electronic health record (EHR) data systems. The proposed model calls for the cost of evidence generation to be shared by manufacturers and payers. Lu brought up the Biologics and Biosimilars Collective Intelligence Consortium (BBCIC) as an example of a comparable model that could provide information and lessons learned.[1] The BBCIC is a nonprofit, collaborative, scientific public service initiative intended to address post-market evidence generation needs for novel biologics, biosimilars, and related products. The proposed model for rapid generation of clinical utility evidence for genomic tests is not the same as the Centers for Medicare & Medicaid Services's (CMS) Coverage with Evidence Development program, Lu noted, in that the CMS program requires that patients participate in a registry or trial, which is slow with regard to recruitment and subsequent data collection.[2] The proposed model is based on a risk-sharing contract between payers and manufacturers so data collection would happen in real time during clinical practice, not through a study or trial, which is the CMS model.

Stakeholder engagement and endorsement is also an important aspect

---

[1]For more information about the Biologics and Biosimilars Collective Intelligence Consortium, see http://www.bbcic.org (accessed January 19, 2018).

[2]For more information about the Centers for Medicare & Medicaid Services' Coverage with Evidence Development program, see https://www.cms.gov/Medicare/Coverage/Coverage-with-Evidence-Development (accessed January 19, 2018).

of the two other components of the model. For example, reaching a temporary coverage agreement requires collaboration and engagement among stakeholders, including manufacturers, diagnostic companies, clinical laboratories, payers, and employers. Leveraging data networks will require engagement and endorsement by the many data stakeholders, including manufacturers, payers, health care systems, EHR vendors, providers, patients, researchers, and government agencies, Lu said.

Leveraging large existing data networks and analytical toolboxes, such as the U.S. Food and Drug Administration's Sentinel Initiative, which includes 223 million individuals in its dataset, or the National Patient-Centered Clinical Research Network (PCORnet), which includes 10 million individuals in its dataset, would help avoid major limitations of multisite research (time and resources), Lu said. Networks can share infrastructure, data curation, analytics, lessons, software development, and other elements. Each organization could participate in multiple data networks. At the same time, each network would still control the governance and coordination of its data (i.e., they would not be "giving data away").

The structure of a data network—PCORnet, for instance—offers a unique opportunity to create a rapid evidence generation program. PCORnet is an initiative that uses large amounts of health data and patient partnerships to make it faster, easier, and less costly to conduct multi-site clinical research. It is a collaboration consisting of a coordinating center and 35 networks including 13 clinical data research networks, 20 people-powered research networks, and 2 health plan research networks. An evidence-generation program based on a PCORnet-like model might have a coordinating center that would produce a computer or statistical program designed to address a particular research query and send that program to each health system within the participating network, Lu said (see Figure 6-1). The participating systems of the network could then run the program against their own data and return the results to the coordinating center to be aggregated (individual patient information is not shared). While many health care systems have records of genetic testing being done, at present many are missing data about which genetic test was administered and the test results, Lu said. Consortiums (e.g., the IGNITE network described by Orlando in Chapter 4) are working to address this and other challenges, such as the lack of interoperability between EHR systems and other data networks and test results that are not in a readily accessible format.[3] Through leveraging

---

[3]For more information on efforts to capture genetic test results in a structured format in the EHR, see DIGITizE, an action collaborative of the Roundtable on Genomics and Precision Health. More information on DIGITizE can be found at http://www.nationalacademies.org/hmd/Activities/Research/GenomicBasedResearch/Innovation-Collaboratives/EHR.aspx (accessed January 23, 2018).

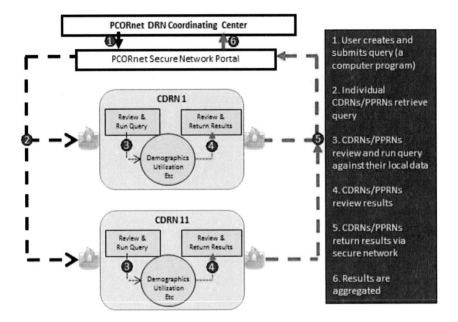

FIGURE 6-1 Example of the evidence-generation model applied in a PCORnet setting.
NOTE: CDRN = clinical data research network; DRN = distributed research network; PPRN = patient-powered research network.
SOURCES: Christine Lu, National Academies of Sciences, Engineering, and Medicine workshop presentation, November 1, 2017, modified from figure presented at PCORnet kick-off meeting, January 21–22, 2014 (slides available at http://www.pcornet.org/wp-content/uploads/2014/02/PCORI-PCORnet-Building-Evidence-Through-Innovation-and-Collaboration-0121141.pdf [accessed March 9, 2018]).

such data networks, Lu concluded, the focus of the model is to capture the missing pieces of genetic test and results data and measure associated patterns of care, clinical outcomes, adverse events, and costs of care in a rapid fashion to generate the clinical and economic utility evidence that is needed to inform clinical practice and policy development.

POLICIES AND INFRASTRUCTURE TO ENABLE THE SHARING OF GENOMIC DATA ACROSS INSTITUTIONS

The policies and infrastructure needed to enable the sharing of genomic data across institutions were discussed by workshop speakers Goddard, Isham, Kho, Leonard, Lu, Murray, and Peterson. Feero also asked them to suggest how the Roundtable could help advance the process of genomic data sharing and contribute to the broader implementation of genomics-based programs in health care systems (see Box 6-1).

As genomic screening programs are implemented across the United States, people will have more enthusiasm for certain kinds of testing, Peterson said. It should be possible to learn from ongoing clinical genetic testing in the community, he said. However, the data that pertain to the results of genetic tests that are being entered into the EHRs are not discrete (i.e., not in a structured format). The data are presumably in a discrete for-

---

BOX 6-1
Areas Highlighted by Individual Speakers That the Roundtable and the Genomics Field Could Explore as a Way to Influence Data Sharing and Foster the Implementation of Genomics-Based Programs

- Incentives for encouraging the harmonization and sharing of genomic and clinical data. (Leonard, Murray)
- Incentives for the entry of discrete data from routine genetic testing into the health system and biorepositories (e.g., depositing into ClinVar or similar data aggregator). (Peterson, Veenstra)
- A common data model for genomics test coding and results. (Goddard, Veenstra)
- Common metrics for assessing health outcomes, cost effectiveness, and other relevant endpoints (e.g., personal utility, family utility). (Leonard)
- Mechanisms for ensuring early engagement, entry, and long-term meaningful participation of typically under-included population groups in developing clinical genomics programs. (Veenstra)
- Health care disparities related to gaining access to necessary genetic testing. (Leonard, Regier)
- Pertinent laws and regulations that might limit the value of genomic medicine outcomes. (Leonard)
- Privacy concerns of participants taking part in genomics-based programs and the technical structures that need to be in place to enable individuals to have a more nuanced consent. (Kho)
- Information about what people and organizations (including employers) value and are willing to pay for with regard to genetic screening. (Kho, Veenstra)
- Areas of tension between the public/population health and genomics research communities about investing in genomics-based programs, given that there may be competing priorities. (Isham)
- Practical financing issues that health care systems are currently struggling with in the mixed payment environment. (Isham)
- Educational approaches to help patients better understand available genetic tests and related downstream treatments. (Isham)

mat on the laboratory testing side, but are not reaching the health system side in that same format. The Roundtable may want to consider how to create incentives for the entry of discrete data from routine testing into the health system and repositories, Peterson said. Such data could be mined for new information about how genomic testing is taking place across the United States and for new genotype–phenotype relationships. One barrier, he suggested, is that institutions are reluctant to invest in ways to receive those data. There are small pilot programs, particularly in academic centers, that integrate data from testing into their health system and data repositories, and the question is how to scale up these models so that this data entry becomes commonplace. Goddard agreed about the need for structured data on whether the test happened *and* what the test result was. These two pieces of information are missing from many existing networks. Work being done by ClinGen on assessing actionability of gene variants is impeded by a lack of consensus in the field on what is meant by actionability, Goddard noted.

There are many challenges involved in capturing information from a genomic test, including the test results, and use of subsequent health care services, Lu said. Further complicating the situation is the fact that there are many different products in use. For example, there are a variety of different panels and sequencing approaches that include the *BRCA* genes, making comparisons challenging. She also said that gathering clinical utility data from a global payment system could be challenging because many items are lumped into one billing code. It might not be possible to discern what kind of test was done or what services were utilized, because the tests and services would be consolidated into a code for cancer care, for example. In response, Leonard said that in a global payment system like the one at the University of Vermont, payment codes would still be tracked, but they would not be submitted to payers.

Leonard proposed several potential activities for the Roundtable to explore. The information needed for analyzing health outcomes and cost effectiveness is not well defined, and Leonard suggested convening a workgroup to define the data and metrics needed for the assessment of health outcomes, cost effectiveness, and other relevant outcomes such as personal utility and family utility. Once the data needed are defined, another workgroup could discuss how best to aggregate the data. Leonard suggested that this process could be informed by groups that are already aggregating data (e.g., PCORnet, HealthConnect, ClinGen, GenomeConnect, Vizient). Finally, she suggested that the Roundtable explore the laws and regulations that might limit the value of genomic medicine outcomes. The Health Insurance Portability and Accountability Act (HIPAA) of 1996, for example, could potentially limit cascade communications with, and testing of, at-risk family members. In addition, there are many individuals who fear potential repercussions from genomic testing, and the Genetic Information Nondiscrimination Act (GINA) of 2008 does not provide full protection from discrimination under all scenarios (i.e., discrimination related to schools, mortgage lending, housing, or life insurance).

The Roundtable could focus on defining what the highest value types of data are, Kho said. Another potential issue for the Roundtable to explore is examining what is needed for a more nuanced consent process, including addressing privacy concerns, and considering the technical structures that would need to be in place to enable individuals to have a more nuanced consent. Finally, Kho said, data sharing is in many ways an economic or value issue. There are opportunities to conduct natural experiments in places where genomic testing is already taking place and to collect information on what people value and are willing to pay for.

Regarding data harmonization and evidence sharing, Murray emphasized the need to motivate the for-profit genomic medicine industry to share its data as they are developed. He suggested that the Roundtable consider how the industry could be incentivized to do so. Another issue for consideration is the need for data standards around penetrance. Currently, Murray observed, if someone has an incidental finding for a monogenic disease, different practitioners around the country would provide different follow-up evaluations. There is also a need to better understand the performance characteristics of phenotyping, he noted. EHR phenotyping has an uncertain negative predictive value, he said, particularly for some genomic conditions. Just because something is not in the EHR does not mean it is not a medical problem for the patient. Self-reporting of data varies according to patients' perspectives, and the data quality and performance characteristics of expert evaluation are also unknown.

The issue of total health care costs was raised as Isham commented on the temporary coverage provision in the model discussed by Lu. There is tremendous chaos and pressure in the larger health system, Isham said, and the total cost of care is driving a lack of investment in other elements critical to health, such as education and economic development. The Roundtable may want to explore some of the tensions between the public–population health perspective and the genomic research perspective, he suggested. He also noted concern about training and the consistency of process outside of the research setting, and he highlighted the opportunity to discuss point-of-care algorithms and tools for helping patients understand the available treatments and courses of action. Another potential topic for Roundtable discussion, Isham suggested, would be practical financing, taking into account the real-world issues that health care systems are struggling with in the current mixed payment environment (i.e., fee-for-service, aggregate payment). More discussion on patient experience and attitudes would also be beneficial, he added.

POTENTIAL ACTION STEPS FOR THOSE IMPLEMENTING GENOMIC SCREENING PROGRAMS

Drawing from the presentations and panel discussions, workshop co-chairs Feero and Veenstra summarized the key messages that individual speakers delivered on the topics of evidence generation, genomic screening programs, and data sharing, and they highlighted some considerations for organizations that are thinking about implementing genomic screening programs. The field of genomics has come a long way in terms of understanding the systematic clinical integration of genomic information, Feero said, and a decade ago much of what has been achieved would have been incomprehensible; however, there are many evidence gaps that still need to be filled.

Considerations from Individual Speakers and Presented in Summary

Generating Evidence

The genomics field is still very much in the evidence-generation stage, Feero said, as opposed to being at the stage of broad implementation of applications with proven benefit. Clinical utility data will be important for facilitating the broader adoption of genomic medicine and the incorporation of genomic data as a routine component of care. Collecting data on personal utility (the amount of usefulness or benefit one can derive from a particular activity) or disutility (harmful or adverse effects associated with a particular activity) will also be very important, Feero said. Without this type of information, the field risks medical misadventures that may be very difficult to recover from, he said. As was emphasized in the discussions, it is important that any population screening program make a clear distinction between research and clinically proven interventions.

Engaging with Populations for Screening

Identifying and meaningfully engaging with typically under-included populations when developing genomics programs is important, Veenstra said, and there is an opportunity to disseminate tools and best practices for researchers interested in engaging diverse populations. Engagement is an ongoing activity throughout the process of genomic screening, and better engagement would help to determine the utility that meets the needs of a given population. Active management of inclusiveness is also important, he said. Enlisting participants from diverse backgrounds (racial/ethnic, socio-economic) will help ensure that accurate knowledge is gained from genomic screening programs, such as data on the clinical utility of genomic tests for all segments of the population.

Facilitating Data Sharing

It is critical that data sharing be advanced, Feero said, as most systems will not have sufficient sample sizes to answer the questions posed. Significant infrastructure, including common data models, needs to be developed in order to fully realize effective data sharing, Veenstra said. There are existing models for data sharing that might be adaptable for genomics-based programs. Some examples discussed were from genomics discovery science, and perhaps these models could be extended and leveraged to help answer questions concerning the integration of genomic screening into health care. It is not yet clear what data should be shared, or how, so in the near term efforts are needed to establish an agreement about what data (outcomes, metrics) need to be collected and shared, Veenstra said. Leonard suggested that the Roundtable could play a role in facilitating the discussion around defining data needs. For the longer term, Veenstra said, there will be a need to engage key decision makers to understand their evidence needs related to the value of genomics-based programs and to create incentives for participation in data sharing.

Designing the Approach

Care is needed in considering what technologies to adopt, what to test for, and how to report that information and for how long, Feero said. Smaller, high-yield panels based on population prevalence may be of more benefit than larger panels with much lower prevalence. Managing expectations is also very important. This includes making sure people understand that a negative result does not necessarily mean they do not have a pathogenic variant, especially if there is a strong family history. A multidisciplinary approach is needed, Feero said, and discipline-specific resources and additional support should be given to non-genetics providers to help them improve the care for patients they see who carry potentially harmful genetic variants (as opposed to getting non-genetics providers to adopt the geneticist perspective on the topic). Research teams should be integrated with programs that are more clinically oriented, Feero said. Early modifications to a study or program design could allow for the ability to answer more questions.

Developing Outcomes to Measure

When developing outcomes for a genomics-based program, Feero said, one should purposefully select outcomes and metrics and evaluate longitudinally and at different intervals in order to inform decisions about whether or not to continue. The outcomes being measured should not be limited to traditional trial metrics (e.g., efficacy), but should include important health-related outcomes more broadly defined, such as personal utility or financial aspects, he said, summarizing concepts discussed by Peterson (see Chapter 3). Electronic infrastructure (particularly the EHR) is lagging and needs attention, he said. When planning the implementation of a genomics program, one should carefully consider the vendor community and how amenable that vendor community will be to genomic testing and genomics data. When a genetic result is returned and an action is taken, it does not necessarily mean that the outcome is related, Feero said. It is important to understand the intermediate steps in order to effect change in the system and potentially improve outcomes.

Improving the Sustainability of Programs

There are multiple pathways by which programs can fund their activities, but long-term financial sustainability is still a work in progress, Feero said. The examples that were discussed at the workshop included a state-funded program, an industry-funded program, a health system–funded program, and federally-funded research. Several speakers noted that organizational leadership buy-in is essential and that organizations should consider evaluating the range of possible ways they could leverage existing systems and resources.

Final Thoughts

One of the major challenges facing the field of genomic medicine, Veenstra said, is how to integrate all of the efforts to collect genomic data that are happening across the United States. Developing a mechanism to bring all the stakeholders together and compile data in a single place to share and learn from will be an ongoing effort. Since its inception, the Roundtable on Genomics and Precision Health has made a great deal of progress in terms of understanding the systematic clinical integration of genomic information; however, Feero said, as the field continues to evolve, there will be new issues to address. Solving these new challenges will take a village, he said, and the Roundtable should continue to bring together all of the relevant stakeholders to identify ways to develop new collaborations, share information, and move the field forward.

References

Bennette, C. S., C. J. Gallego, W. Burke, G. P. Jarvik, and D. L. Veenstra. 2015. The cost-effectiveness of returning incidental findings from next-generation genomic sequencing. *Genetics in Medicine* 17(7):587–595.

Canto, J. G., C. I. Kiefe, W. J. Rogers, E. D. Peterson, P. D. Frederick, W. J. French, C. M. Gibson, C. V. Pollack, Jr., J. P. Ornato, R. J. Zalenski, J. Penney, A. J. Tiefenbrunn, P. Greenland, and NRMI Investigators. 2011. Number of coronary heart disease risk factors and mortality in patients with first myocardial infarction. *JAMA* 306(19):2120–2127.

Carey, D. J., S. N. Fetterolf, F. D. Davis, W. A. Faucett, H. L. Kirchner, U. Mirshahi, M. F. Murray, D. T. Smelser, G. S. Gerhard, and D. H. Ledbetter. 2016. The Geisinger MyCode community health initiative: An electronic health record-linked biobank for precision medicine research. *Genetics in Medicine* 18(9):906–913.

Cavallari, L. H., and M. A. Perera. 2012. The future of warfarin pharmacogenetics in under-represented minority groups. *Future Cardiology* 8(4):563–576.

Chambers, D. A., W. G. Feero, and M. J. Khoury. 2016. Convergence of implementation science, precision medicine, and the learning health care system: A new model for biomedical research. *JAMA* 315(18):1941–1942.

Damschroder, L. J., D. C. Aron, R. E. Keith, S. R. Kirsh, J. A. Alexander, and J. C. Lowery. 2009. Fostering implementation of health services research findings into practice: A consolidated framework for advancing implementation science. *Implementation Science* 4:50.

Dewey, F. E., V. Gusarova, C. O'Dushlaine, O. Gottesman, J. Trejos, C. Hunt, C. V. Van Hout, L. Habegger, D. Buckler, K. M. Lai, J. B. Leader, M. F. Murray, M. D. Ritchie, H. L. Kirchner, D. H. Ledbetter, J. Penn, A. Lopez, I. B. Borecki, J. D. Overton, J. G. Reid, D. J. Carey, A. J. Murphy, G. D. Yancopoulos, A. Baras, J. Gromada, and A. R. Shuldiner. 2016. Inactivating variants in *ANGPTL4* and risk of coronary artery disease. *New England Journal of Medicine* 374(12):1123–1133.

Dotson, W. D., M. P. Douglas, K. Kolor, A. C. Stewart, M. S. Bowen, M. Gwinn, A. Wulf, H. M. Anders, C. Q. Chang, M. Clyne, T. K. Lam, S. D. Schully, M. Marrone, W. G. Feero, and M. J. Khoury. 2014. Prioritizing genomic applications for action by level of evidence: A horizon-scanning method. *Clinical Pharmacology & Therapeutics* 95(4): 394–402.

Foster, M. W., J. J. Mulvihill, and R. R. Sharp. 2009. Evaluating the utility of personal genomic information. *Genetics in Medicine* 11(8):570–574.

Gage, B. F., A. R. Bass, H. Lin, S. C. Woller, S. M. Stevens, N. Al-Hammadi, J. Li, T. Rodriguez, Jr., J. P. Miller, G. A. McMillin, R. C. Pendleton, A. K. Jaffer, C. R. King, B. DeVore Whipple, R. Porche-Sorbet, L. Napoli, K. Merritt, A. M. Thompson, G. Hyun, J. L. Anderson, W. Hollomon, R. L. Barrack, R. M. Nunley, G. Moskowitz, V. Davila-Roman, and C. S. Eby. 2017. Effect of genotype-guided warfarin dosing on clinical events and anticoagulation control among patients undergoing hip or knee arthroplasty. The GIFT randomized control trial. *JAMA* 318(12):1115–1124.

Genovese, G., D. J. Friedman, M. D. Ross, L. Lecordier, P. Uzureau, B. I. Freedman, D. W. Bowden, C. D. Langefeld, T. K. Oleksyk, A. L. Uscinski Knob, A. J. Bernhardy, P. J. Hicks, G. W. Nelson, B. Vanhollebeke, C. A. Winkler, J. B. Kopp, E. Pays, and M. R. Pollak. 2010. Association of trypanolytic APOL1 variants with kidney disease in African Americans. *Science* 329(5993):841–845.

Graves, J. A., S. Garbett, Z. Zhou, and J. Peterson. 2017. The value of pharmacogenomic information. NBER Working Paper 24134. http://www.nber.org/papers/w24134.pdf (accessed March 9, 2018).

Green, L. A., G. E. Fryer, Jr., B. P. Yawn, D. Lanier, and S. M. Dovey. 2001. The ecology of medical care revisited. *New England Journal of Medicine* 344(26):2021–2025.

Green, R. C., J. S. Berg, W. W. Grody, S. S. Kalia, B. R. Korf, C. L. Martin, and L. G. Biesecker. 2013. ACMG recommendations for reporting of incidental findings in clinical exome and genome sequencing. *Genetics in Medicine* 15(7):565–574.

Griffiths, A. J. F., J. H. Miller, D. T. Suzuki, R. C. Lewontin, and W. M. Gelbart. 2000. Penetrance and expressivity. *An introduction to genetic analysis, 7th edition.* New York: W.H. Freeman. https://www.ncbi.nlm.nih.gov/books/NBK22090 (accessed March 9, 2018).

Grosse, S. D., L. Kalman, and M. J. Khoury. 2010. Evaluation of the validity and utility of genetic testing for rare diseases. *Advances in Experimental Medicine and Biology* 686:115–131.

Horowitz, C. R., K. Ferryman, R. Negron, T. Sabin, M. Rodriguez, R. F. Zinberg, E. Böttinger, and M. Robinson. 2017. Race, genomics and chronic disease: What patients with African ancestry have to say. *Journal of Health Care for the Poor and Underserved* 28(1): 248–260.

IOM (Institute of Medicine). 2013. *Observational studies in a learning health system: Workshop summary.* Washington, DC: The National Academies Press.

IOM. 2015. *Genomics-enabled learning health care systems: Gathering and using genomic information to improve patient care and research: Workshop summary.* Washington, DC: The National Academies Press.

Kalia, S. S., K. Adelman, S. J. Bale, W. K. Chung, C. Eng, J. P. Evans, G. E. Herman, S. B. Hufnagel, T. E. Klein, B. R. Korf, K. D. McKelvey, K. E. Ormond, C. S. Richards, C. N. Vlangos, M. Watson, C. L. Martin, and D. T. Miller. 2017. Recommendations for reporting of secondary findings in clinical exome and genome sequencing, 2016 update (ACMG SF v2.0): A policy statement of the American College of Medical Genetics and Genomics. *Genetics in Medicine* 19(2):249–255.

Kaplan, B., C. Caddle-Steele, G. Chisholm, W. A. Esmond, K. Ferryman, M. Gertner, C. Goytia, D. Hauser, L. D. Richardson, M. Robinson, and C. R. Horowitz. 2017. A culture of understanding: Reflections and suggestions from a genomics research community board. *Progress in Community Health Partnerships* 11(2):161–165.

Khera, A. V., H. H. Won, G. M. Peloso, K. S. Lawson, T. M. Bartz, X. Deng, E. M. van Leeuwen, P. Natarajan, C. A. Emdin, A. G. Bick, A. C. Morrison, J. A. Brody, N. Gupta, A. Nomura, T. Kessler, S. Duga, J. C. Bis, C. M. van Duijn, L. A. Cupples, B. Psaty, D. J. Rader, J. Danesh, H. Schunkert, R. McPherson, M. Farrall, H. Watkins, E. Lander, J. G. Wilson, A. Correa, E. Boerwinkle, P. A. Merlini, D. Ardissino, D. Saleheen, S. Gabriel, and S. Kathiresan. 2016. Diagnostic yield and clinical utility of sequencing familial hypercholesterolemia genes in patients with severe hypercholesterolemia. *Journal of the American College of Cardiology* 67(22):2578–2589.

Kho, A. N., J. P. Cashy, K. L. Jackson, A. R. Pah, S. Goel, J. Boehnke, J. E. Humphries, S. D. Kominers, B. N. Hota, S. A. Sims, B. A. Malin, D. D. French, T. L. Walunas, D. O. Meltzer, E. O. Kaleba, R. C. Jones, and W. L. Galanter. 2015. Design and implementation of a privacy protecting electronic health record linkage tool in Chicago. *Journal of the American Medical Informatics Association* 22(5):1072–1080.

Kimmel, S. E., B. French, S. E. Kasner, J. A. Johnson, J. L. Anderson, B. F. Gage, Y. D. Rosenberg, C. S. Eby, R. A. Madigan, R. B. McBane, S. Z. Abdel-Rahman, S. M. Stevens, S. Yale, E. R. Mohler 3rd, M. C. Fang, V. Shah, R. B. Horenstein, N. A. Limdi, J. A. Muldowney 3rd, J. Gujral, P. Delafontaine, R. J. Desnick, T. L. Ortel, H. H. Billett, R. C. Pendleton, N. L. Geller, J. L. Halperin, S. Z. Goldhaber, M. D. Caldwell, R. M. Califf, and J. H. Ellenberg; for the COAG Investigators. 2013. A pharmacogenetic versus a clinical algorithm for warfarin dosing. *New England Journal of Medicine* 369(24):2283–2293.

Knight, S. J., A. F. Mohamed, D. A. Marshall, U. Ladabaum, K. A. Phillips, and J. M. Walsh. 2015. Value of genetic testing for hereditary colorectal cancer in a probability-based U.S. online sample. *Medical Decision Making* 35(6):734–744.

Kraft, S. A., J. L. Schneider, M. C. Leo, T. L. Kauffman, J. V. Davis, K. M. Porter, C. K. McMullen, B. S. Wilfond, and K. A. B. Goddard. 2018. Patient actions and reactions after receiving negative results from expanded carrier screening. *Clinical Genetics.* January 2. doi: 10.1111/cge.13206. [Epub ahead of print]. https://www.ncbi.nlm.nih.gov/pubmed/29293279 (accessed March 9, 2018).

Lancsar, E., and J. Louviere. 2008. Conducting discrete choice experiments to inform health-care decision making. *Pharmacoeconomics* 26:661–677.

Lu, C. Y., M. S. Williams, G. S. Ginsburg, S. Toh, J. S. Brown, and M. J. Khoury. 2017. A proposed approach to accelerate evidence generation for genomics-based technologies in the context of a learning health system. *Genetics in Medicine* August 10. doi: 10.1038/gim.2017.122. [Epub ahead of print]. https://www.ncbi.nlm.nih.gov/pubmed/28796238 (accessed March 9, 2018).

Marshall, D. A., J. M. Gonzalez, K. V. MacDonald, and F. R. Johnson. 2017. Estimating preferences for complex health technologies: Lessons learned and implications for personalized medicine. *Value in Health* 20(1):32–39.

McFadden, D. 1974. Conditional logit analysis of qualitative choice behavior. In *Frontiers in econometrics*, edited by P. Zarembka. New York: Academic Press. Pp. 105–142.

NASEM (National Academies of Sciences, Engineering, and Medicine). 2016. *Applying an implementation science approach to genomic medicine: Workshop summary.* Washington, DC: The National Academies Press.

Neumann, P., G. D. Sanders, L. B. Russell, J. E. Siegel, and T. G. Ganiats. 2017. *Cost-effectiveness in health and medicine: 2nd edition.* New York: Oxford University Press.

NIDDK (National Institute of Diabetes and Digestive and Kidney Diseases). 2016. *Kidney disease statistics for the United States.* https://www.niddk.nih.gov/health-information/health-statistics/kidney-disease (accessed January 24, 2018).

NIMH (National Institute of Mental Health). 2017. *What is prevalence?* https://www.nimh.nih.gov/health/statistics/prevalence/index.shtml (accessed January 22, 2018).

Orlando, L. A., N. R. Sperber, C. Voils, M. Nichols, R. A. Myers, R. R. Wu, T. Rakhra-Burris, K. D. Levy, M. Levy, T. I. Pollin, Y. Guan, C. R. Horowitz, M. Ramos, S. E. Kimmel, C. W. McDonough, E. B. Madden, and L. J. Damschroder. 2017. Developing a common framework for evaluating the implementation of genomic medicine interventions in clinical care: The IGNITE Network's Common Measures Working Group. *Genetics in Medicine* September 14. [Epub ahead of print]. https://www.ncbi.nlm.nih.gov/pubmed/28914267 (accessed March 9, 2018).

Peterson, J., J. Field, K. Unertl, J. Schildcrout, D. Johnson, Y. Shi, I. Danciu, J. Cleator, J. Pulley, J. McPherson, J. Denny, M. Laposata, D. Roden, and K. Johnson. 2016. Physician response to implementation of genotype-tailored antiplatelet therapy. *Clinical Pharmacology & Therapeutics* 100:67–74.

Phillips, K. A., P. A. Deverka, H. C. Sox, M. J. Khoury, L. G. Sandy, G. S. Ginsburg, S. R. Tunis, L. A. Orlando, and M. P. Douglas. 2017. Making genomic medicine evidence-based and patient-centered: A structured review and landscape analysis of comparative effectiveness research. *Genetics in Medicine* 19(10):1081–1091.

Pirmohamed, M., G. Burnside, N. Eriksson, A. L. Jorgensen, C. H. Toh, T. Nicholson, P. Kesteven, C. Christersson, B. Wahlström, C. Stafberg, J. E. Zhang, H. Leathart, H. Kohnke, A. H. Maitland-van der Zee, P. R. Williamson, A. K. Daly, P. Avery, F. Kamali, and M. Wadelius, for the EU-PACT Group. 2013. A randomized trial of genotype-guided dosing of warfarin. *New England Journal of Medicine* 369(24):2294–2303.

Plon, S. E., D. M. Eccles, D. Easton, W. D. Foulkes, M. Genuardi, M. S. Greenblatt, and S. Tavtigian. 2008. Sequence variant classification and reporting: Recommendations for improving the interpretation of cancer susceptibility genetic test results. *Human Mutation* 29(11):1282–1291.

Powell, C. 2016. Presentation at the Advisory Committee on Heritable Disorders in Newborns and Children. August 25. https://www.hrsa.gov/sites/default/files/hrsa/advisory-committees/heritable-disorders/meetings/20160825/powell.pdf (accessed March 9, 2018).

Regier, D. A., J. M. Friedman, N. Makela, M. Ryan, and C. A. Marra. 2009. Valuing the benefit of diagnostic testing for genetic causes of idiopathic developmental disability: Willingness to pay from families of affected children. *Clinical Genetics* 75(6):514–521.

Regier, D. A., S. J. Peacock, R. Pataky, K. van der Hoek, G. Jarvik, and D. A. Veenstra. 2015. Societal preferences for the return of incidental findings from clinical genomic sequencing: A discrete choice experiment. *CMAJ* 187(6):E190–E197.

Rehm, H. L., J. S. Berg, L. D. Brooks, C. D. Bustamante, J. P. Evans, M. J. Landrum, D. H. Ledbetter, D. R. Maglott, C. L. Martin, R. L. Nussbaum, S. E. Plon, E. M. Ramos, S. T. Sherry, and M. S. Watson for ClinGen. 2015. ClinGen—The clinical genome resource. *New England Journal of Medicine* 372(23):2235–2242.

Richards, S., N. Aziz, S. Bale, D. Bick, S. Das, J. Gastier-Foster, W. W. Grody, M. Hegde, E. Lyon, E. Spector, K. Voelkerding, and H. L. Rehm, on behalf of the ACMG Laboratory Quality Assurance Committee. 2015. Standards and guidelines for the interpretation of sequence variants: A joint consensus recommendation of the American College of Medical Genetics and Genomics and the Association for Molecular Pathology. *Genetics in Medicine* 17(5):405–424.

Roberts, M. C., M. Clyne, A. E. Kennedy, D. A. Chambers, and M. J. Khoury. 2017. The current state of funded NIH grants in implementation science in genomic medicine: A portfolio analysis. *Genetics in Medicine* Oct 26. doi: 10.1038/gim.2017.180. [Epub ahead of print]. https://www.nature.com/articles/gim2017180 (accessed March 9, 2018).

Ross, L. F., H. M. Saal, K. L. David, R. R. Anderson, the American Academy of Pediatrics, and the American College of Medical Genetics and Genomics. 2013. Technical report: Ethical and policy issues in genetic testing and screening of children. *Genetics in Medicine* 15(3):234–245.

Rothstein, M. A. 2005. Genetic exceptionalism & legislative pragmatism. *Hastings Center Report* 35(4):27–33. https://muse.jhu.edu (accessed January 18, 2018).

Sperber, N. R., S. M. Andrews, C. I. Voils, G. L. Green, D. Provenzale, and S. Knight. 2016. Barriers and facilitators to adoption of genomic services for colorectal care within the Veterans Health Administration. *Journal of Personal Medicine* 6(2):16.

Trivedi, B. P. 2017. Medicine's future? *Science* 358(6362):436–440.

Verhoef, T. I., W. K. Redekop, S. Langenskiold, F. Kamali, M. Wadelius, G. Burnside, A. H. Maitland-van der Zee, D. A. Hughes, and M. Pirmohamed. 2016. Cost-effectiveness of pharmacogenetic-guided dosing of warfarin in the United Kingdom and Sweden. *Pharmacogenomics Journal* 16(5):478–484.

Walsh, J., M. Arora, C. Hosenfeld, U. Ladabaum, M. Kuppermann, and S. J. Knight. 2012. Preferences for genetic testing to identify hereditary colorectal cancer: Perspectives of high-risk patients, community members, and clinicians. *Journal of Cancer Education* 27(1):112–119.

Wilson, J. M. G., and G. Jungner. 1968. *Principles and practice of screening for disease.* Geneva: World Health Organization.

Appendix A

Workshop Agenda

Implementing and Evaluating Genomic Screening Programs
in Health Care Systems:
A Workshop
November 1, 2017

The Keck Center of the National Academies, Room 100
500 Fifth Street, NW
Washington, DC 20001

BACKGROUND

Genomic applications can be embedded into a broad range of clinical and research activities. Increasing amounts of genomic data are currently being generated and incorporated into a variety of health care systems[1] in the United States and abroad, and each instance presents a natural "experiment" offering the opportunity for learning about the integration of genomics into health care ecosystems. Of particular interest is genomic screening or **genomics-based screening programs,** referred to in the context of this workshop as clinical screening programs with the goal of examining genes or variants in unselected populations in order to identify individuals at risk for future disease or adverse drug outcomes for which there are clinical actions to mitigate risk. Many current genomics-based screening programs examine germline variability in specific genes that have been evaluated and recommended by groups such as the American College of Medical Genetics and Genomics, U.S. Preventive Services Task Force, or Evaluation of Genomics Applications in Practice and Prevention. There is potential strength in evaluating common outcomes of implementing these screening programs across multiple large health care systems and organizations that incorporate data from diverse population groups in order to

---

[1]For the purposes of this workshop, *health systems* are referred to as entities providing medical care to a select population. Examples may include a for-profit or nonprofit health care delivery system or a public health system.

understand how genomics may or may not ultimately benefit all population groups. Tracking data from early implementers on the potential health
benefits and harms of genomic screening programs may provide important
evidence needed to assess the effectiveness and safety of genomic screening
in unselected populations.[2]

AGENDA

8:30 a.m.   **Opening Remarks**

GEOFFREY GINSBURG, *Roundtable Co-Chair*
Director, Duke Center for Applied Genomics & Precision
Medicine
Professor, Medicine, Pathology, and Biomedical
Engineering
Duke University Medical Center

8:35 a.m.   **Charge to Workshop Speakers and Participants**

W. GREGORY FEERO, *Workshop Co-Chair*
Associate Editor, *Journal of the American Medical
Association*
Faculty
Maine Dartmouth Family Medicine Residency Program

DAVID VEENSTRA, *Workshop Co-Chair*
Professor and Associate Director
Pharmaceutical Outcomes Research and Policy Program
University of Washington, Seattle

8:50 a.m.   **Keynote Lecture**

MICHAEL MURRAY
Director of Clinical Genomics
Geisinger Health System

9:10 a.m.   **Clarifying Questions from Workshop Participants**

---

[2]The term *population* in the context of this workshop refers to individuals in the context of
a health system that has implemented or is planning to implement a genomics-based screening program.

SESSION I: EVIDENCE CONSIDERATIONS FOR INTEGRATING GENOMICS-BASED PROGRAMS INTO HEALTH SYSTEMS

Session Objective:

- To examine the types of clinical data and other evidence that are currently being collected by genomics-based programs at health systems and to consider opportunities for advancing knowledge of clinical utility.

Key Questions:

- What evidence will your program generate, and how will it be useful in the future in terms of evaluating the value and utility of these activities?
- Are you currently sharing information from your genomics-based program or data across systems or organizations? How and with whom?
- What outcomes are important for genomics-based programs to measure? What potential impacts are there on care when deciding to invest in genomics-based programs?
- If you run into challenges such as a lack of evidence of utility or any harms (e.g., privacy, discrimination) to participants from implementing a genetic test in your program, how do you plan to track these outcomes and address them?

Session Moderator: George Isham, Senior Advisor, HealthPartners

9:20 a.m.	KATRINA GODDARD Senior Investigator Kaiser Permanente Center for Health Research
9:35 a.m.	BRUCE KORF Wayne H. and Sara Crews Finley Chair in Medical Genetics Professor and Chair, Department of Genetics Director, Heflin Center for Genomic Sciences University of Alabama at Birmingham School of Medicine
9:50 a.m.	DEBRA LEONARD Chair of Pathology and Laboratory Medicine University of Vermont Medical Center

10:05 a.m.   **Panel Discussion with Speakers and Workshop
                  Participants**
                  KATRINA GODDARD, BRUCE KORF, DEBRA LEONARD,
                  MICHAEL MURRAY

10:35 a.m.   **Break**

SESSION II: FINANCIAL CONSIDERATIONS FOR IMPLEMENTING GENOMICS-BASED SCREENING PROGRAMS

Session Objectives:

- To discuss the financial considerations associated with genomics-based programs, including
  o Available models that can effectively evaluate genomics-based programs and the value they represent to their institution;
  o Approaches to measuring return on investment from implementation of genomics-based screening programs; and
  o Best practices for data sharing related to economic evaluations of genomics-based programs.

Key Questions:

- What business models are available to fund genomics-based screening programs? Would this program remain a priority for your organization if the current source of funding was no longer available? Is the program built to be sustainable? How?
- Are genomics-based programs affordable? Do they provide clinical utility or other value that can justify implementing the program? Beyond the cost of the genetic test itself, what are the downstream costs of care that need to be taken into account?
- How can institutions evaluate the opportunity costs associated with genomics implementation into a health system?
- Are there models that support data sharing between individual health care systems that are implementing genomics-based programs?
- What challenges do these programs create for clinical workflow?

Session Moderator: David Veenstra, Professor and Associate Director of Pharmaceutical Outcomes Research and Policy Program, Department of Pharmacy, University of Washington, Seattle

10:50 a.m.	BRADFORD POWELL Clinical Assistant Professor Department of Genetics University of North Carolina at Chapel Hill
11:05 a.m.	JOSH PETERSON Associate Professor of Biomedical Informatics and Medicine Vanderbilt University Medical Center
11:20 a.m.	DEAN REGIER Assistant Professor, School of Population and Public Health University of British Columbia
11:35 a.m.	**Panel Discussion with Speakers and Audience Members**
12:05 p.m.	**Working Lunch**

SESSION III: CONSIDERING APPROACHES TO OPTIMIZE DATA SHARING AMONG EARLY IMPLEMENTERS OF GENOMICS-BASED PROGRAMS

Session Objective:

- To explore new ideas and opportunities for collaborative networks as a way for sharing economic and clinical outcome data about genomics-based programs between and within large-scale health care organizations.

Key Questions:

- How could data sharing across systems and organizations affect the measurement of value and clinical utility of genomics-based programs?
- Are there incentives for overcoming cultural and technological barriers to sharing data across systems and organizations? What are the incentives? If they do not exist, what is needed?
- What common outcomes or endpoints would be useful to collect from early implementers of genomics-based programs? What are the ideal data elements that should be collected from genomics-based programs?

Session Moderator: Marc Grodman, Assistant Professor of Clinical Medicine, Columbia University

1:05 p.m.	REX CHISHOLM Vice Dean, Scientific Affairs and Graduate Education Adam and Richard T. Lind Professor of Medical Genetics Northwestern University
1:20 p.m.	ERIC BOERWINKLE Dean and M. David Low Chair in Public Health Kozmetsky Family Chair in Human Genetics University of Texas Health Science Center at Houston
1:35 p.m.	RICHARD TURNER Clinical Research Fellow in Clinical Pharmacology and Therapeutics Royal Liverpool University Hospital and University of Liverpool
1:50 p.m.	LORI ORLANDO Associate Professor of Medicine Duke University School of Medicine
2:05 p.m.	**Panel Discussion with Speakers and Workshop Participants**
2:35 p.m.	**Break**

SESSION IV: WORKING TOWARD THE NEEDS OF PARTICIPANTS AND IMPROVING DIVERSITY AND EQUITY

Session Objective:

- To consider policy issues associated with implementation of genomics-based programs in health systems and potentially in public health, including
  o Approaches to ensuring data security and participant privacy and
  o Methods for ensuring that genomics-based programs are accessible to a diverse group of participants.

Key Questions:

- Is this the right time to be studying use of genomic data and population health management in health systems? Why?
- How can genomics-based programs be designed in such a way to reach a diverse group of participants?
- How can genomics-based programs be equitably distributed regardless of educational status, income level, ethnicity, or other variables?
- If the early evidence indicates that genomics-based programs do not provide value and utility (and potentially demonstrate harms to participants), are the programs discontinued? How are they de-implemented and/or assessed again at a later date?

Session Moderator: Vence Bonham, Senior Advisor to the National Human Genome Research Institute Director on Genomics and Health Disparities, National Human Genome Research Institute, National Institutes of Health

2:50 p.m.	SARA KNIGHT Professor, Division of Preventive Medicine, School of Medicine University of Alabama at Birmingham
3:05 p.m.	CAROL HOROWITZ Professor, Population Health Science and Policy Mount Sinai Hospital
3:20 p.m.	ABEL KHO Director, Center for Health Information Partnerships Northwestern University
3:35 p.m.	**Panel Discussion with Speakers and Workshop Participants**

SESSION V: NEXT STEPS TOWARD IMPROVING HEALTH THROUGH THE INTEGRATION OF GENOMICS-BASED PROGRAMS

Session Objectives:

- To discuss ideas for actionable next steps that could support the implementation of genomics-based programs in health systems.

- To consider infrastructure and resources that are needed to share data collected in clinical care across health systems for health outcomes and economics research.

Key Questions:

- Thinking about the workshop discussions today, what would be a game changer in terms of facilitating data sharing among early implementers of genomics-based programs?
- What next steps are critical for building an active learning model for outcome data on benefits, harms, and costs collected in genomics-based programs?

Session Moderator: W. Gregory Feero, Workshop Co-Chair, Faculty, Maine Dartmouth Family Medicine Residency Program

4:05 p.m.	**A Model for Accelerating Evidence Generation for Genomic Technologies in the Context of a Learning Health Care System**
	CHRISTINE LU Associate Professor Department of Population Medicine Harvard Medical School
4:20 p.m.	**Clarifying Questions**
4:30 p.m.	**Final Panel Discussion: What policies and infrastructure need to be in place to enable data sharing across institutions?**
	KATRINA GODDARD GEORGE ISHAM ABEL KHO DEBRA LEONARD MICHAEL MURRAY JOSH PETERSON

5:05 p.m.   **Final Remarks from Workshop Co-Chairs**
                 W. GREGORY FEERO, *Workshop Co-Chair*
                 Associate Editor, *Journal of the American Medical
                 Association*
                 Faculty
                 Maine Dartmouth Family Medicine Residency Program

                 DAVID VEENSTRA, *Workshop Co-Chair*
                 Professor and Associate Director
                 Pharmaceutical Outcomes Research and Policy Program
                 University of Washington, Seattle

5:15 p.m.   **Adjourn**

Appendix B

Speaker Biographies

Eric Boerwinkle, Ph.D., is the dean and M. David Low Chair of Public Health at The University of Texas Health Science Center at Houston (UTHealth) School of Public Health. He began serving as dean on January 1, 2016. Dr. Boerwinkle joined the UTHealth faculty in 1986 and served as chair of the Department of Epidemiology, Human Genetics and Environmental Health at UTHealth School of Public Health from 2003 to 2015. He has also directed the Human Genetics Center at the School of Public Health and the Brown Foundation Institute for Molecular Medicine for the Prevention of Human Diseases, which are a part of UTHealth. He holds the Kozmetsky Family Chair in Human Genetics at the School of Public Health as well.

Author of more than 800 scientific papers, Dr. Boerwinkle has led groundbreaking research on the connection between genes and health. He and his colleagues completed the world's first genome-wide analyses for a variety of cardiovascular disease risk factors, including hypertension and diabetes. These investigations have been a critical step in developing drugs that lower disease risk.

Dr. Boerwinkle earned a Ph.D. in human genetics from the University of Michigan, Ann Arbor, where he also earned master's degrees in human genetics and statistics. In 2003 he was the recipient of the President's Scholar Award, which recognizes distinguished achievements in research and education at UTHealth.

Dr. Boerwinkle has served on several national research panels, including the Advisory Council for the National Human Genome Research Institute and the board of external advisors for the National Heart, Lung, and Blood

Institute, part of the National Institutes of Health. Dr. Boerwinkle has also served as an editor of several journals, including *Circulation*, *Epidemiology*, *Genetic Epidemiology*, and the *American Journal of Epidemiology*.

Rex Chisholm, Ph.D., is the Adam and Richard T. Lind Professor of Medical Genetics in the Feinberg School of Medicine and a professor of cell and molecular biology and surgery. He was the founding director of the Center for Genetic Medicine. Since 2007 he has served as vice dean for scientific affairs in the Feinberg School. In October 2012 he was also appointed associate vice president for research of Northwestern University.

A faculty member at Northwestern University since 1984, Dr. Chisholm is the author of more than 125 scientific publications. His research focuses on genomics and bioinformatics. Dr. Chisholm leads a major DNA biobanking effort at Northwestern University, NUgene. NUgene enrolls research participants in a study focused on investigating the genetic contributions to human disease, therapeutic outcomes, and gene–environment interactions. NUgene is a participant in the National Human Genome Research Institute (NHGRI)-funded eMERGE network (www.gwas.net)—a network of electronic medical record–linked biobanks. The goal of the eMERGE network project is to establish a program for genomics-informed personalized medicine in partnership with Northwestern's health care affiliates. Dr. Chisholm is the principal investigator of dictyBase, the National Institutes of Health (NIH)-funded genome database for the cellular slime mold *Dictyostelium* and is an NHGRI-funded member of the Gene Ontology Consortium. His research has been supported by NIH, the American Cancer Society, the American Heart Association, and the Department of Defense.

Katrina Goddard, Ph.D., is a genetic epidemiologist who focuses on public health genomics and the translation of genetic testing into practice. She joined the Kaiser Permanente Center for Health Research in 2007.

Dr. Goddard has directed or collaborated on more than 20 federally funded research studies. She is the co-principal investigator of a study that is exploring the use of genome sequencing in the clinical context of preconception carrier screening. She also led a project implementing universal tumor screening for Lynch syndrome and a National Cancer Institute (NCI)-funded collaboration to evaluate evidence on breast cancer genomic applications. She was the co-principal investigator of the NCI-funded Grand Opportunity award CERGEN, which evaluated the cost, diffusion, and outcomes of KRAS testing to direct treatment decisions across 11 health care systems. She was also the site principal investigator for the GeneScreen pilot program which explored targeted genomic screening for medically actionable conditions in the adult general population.

Dr. Goddard was the founding director for the NW Biobank. She co-chaired a committee to develop plans for the integration and coordination of biobanking activities across seven Kaiser Permanente regions. This planning led to the launch of the Kaiser Permanente Research Bank in 2014.

Dr. Goddard has contributed to knowledge synthesis products that have far-reaching impact for numerous national organizations. She currently directs the Knowledge Synthesis Team (KST) and co-chairs the Actionability Work Group for the ClinGen Consortium. The KST provides systematic evidence summaries on the ClinGen website for the entire genomics community.

Prior to her appointment as a senior investigator, Dr. Goddard was on the faculty at Case Western Reserve University in the Division of Genetic and Molecular Epidemiology. She was involved in several large-scale gene discovery projects there and was associate director of the Human Genetic Analysis Resource. She received her Ph.D. in biostatistics from the University of Washington and a B.S. in molecular biology from the University of Wisconsin–Madison.

Carol R. Horowitz, M.D., M.P.H., is a practicing general internist in Harlem and a health services researcher and professor in the Department of Population Health Science and Policy Department of Medicine at Mount Sinai. She uses community- and stakeholder-engaged approaches to understand and eliminate health disparities related to common chronic diseases. She co-directs Mount Sinai's Center for Health Equity and Community Engaged Research, the Sinai Clinical and Translational Science Award's Community Engaged Research Core; has been a principal investigator and investigator on numerous National Institutes of Health, the Centers for Disease Control and Research, and Patient-Centered Outcomes Research Institute (PCORI) grants related to chronic disease prevention and control; directs stakeholder engagement for the PCORI-funded New York City Clinical Data Research Network and chaired NHGRI's translational genomics consortium, IGNITE, and co-chairs NHGRI's CSER2 consortium. Dr. Horowitz has implemented and evaluated programs to improve the quality of care and the outcomes of diverse populations of adults with diabetes, obesity, cardiovascular disease, and other health conditions through clinical and community programs. She has extensive experience in multi-method (quantitative and qualitative) research, clinical research training, program and intervention development, conducting and analyzing multi-site randomized trials, and managing and working with large, transdisciplinary teams that include diverse researchers, patients, clinicians, advocates, and entrepreneurs and policy makers. She mentors students, residents, fellows, and junior faculty; serves on community boards; and is active in her local community. She has received numerous honors, including a special award from the Department of Health and Human Services for Excellence in Contributions to Diabetes and the Rudin New York City Prize for Medicine and Health. Dr. Horowitz received her M.D. from Cornell University and her primary care training at Albert Einstein, and she received an M.P.H. at the University of Washington as a Robert Wood Johnson Foundation Clinical Scholar.

George Isham, M.D., is a senior advisor at HealthPartners in Minneapolis, Minnesota. As a senior advisor, Dr. Isham is responsible for working with the board of directors and the senior management team of HealthPartners on health and quality of care improvement for patients, members, and the community. Prior to his appointment as a senior advisor in 2012, Dr. Isham served as HealthPartners' medical director and chief health officer, a position he had held since 1993. Dr. Isham is also a senior fellow at the HealthPartners Institute for Education and Research. As a senior fellow, he is responsible for facilitating forward progress at the intersection of population health research and public policy.

Dr. Isham is an elected member of the National Academy of Medicine and was designated as a national associate of the Institute of Medicine in 2003 in recognition of his contribution to its work. He is active in health policy nationally and currently co-chairs the National Academies of Sciences, Engineering, and Medicine's Roundtable on Population Health Improvement. He is a former member of the Centers for Disease Control and Prevention's Task Force on Community Preventive Services and the Agency for Healthcare Research and Quality's U.S. Preventive Services Task Force, the founding co-chair of the National Committee for Quality Assurance's committee on performance measurement, the founding co-chair of the National Quality Forum's Measurement Application Partnership, and a founding member of the advisory board for the National Guideline Clearinghouse.

Dr. Isham completed his bachelor of arts degree in zoology and a master of science degree in preventive medicine/administrative medicine at the University of Wisconsin–Madison and his doctor of medicine degree from the University of Illinois, following which he completed his internship and residency in internal medicine at the University of Wisconsin Hospital and Clinics, in Madison, Wisconsin.

Abel Kho, Ph.D., is an associate professor of medicine and preventive medicine in the Feinberg School of Medicine at Northwestern University and the director of the Center for Health Information Partnerships within the Institute for Public Health and Medicine. His research focuses on developing regional electronic health record (EHR)-enabled data sharing platforms for a range of health applications, including tracking drug-resistant infections and estimating population-level disease burden. Dr. Kho is a co-principal investigator and the informatics lead of the Chicago Area Patient Centered Outcomes Research Network (PCORnet), one of the Patient-Centered Outcomes Research Institute–funded clinical data research networks and also serves as a co-chair of the Data Standards, Security and Network Infrastructure Task Force of PCORnet. As a member of the eMERGE (Electronic Medical Records and Genomics) consortium, he has developed EHR-based phenotyping methods to enable high-throughput genetic studies. He maintains an active primary care practice, which guides his role as the principal investigator of the Chicago Health IT Regional Extension Center, which assists primary care practices in Chicago to achieve meaningful use of EHRs, and also guides his role leading Illinois' involvement in the Centers for Medicare & Medicaid Services–sponsored Great Lakes Practice Transformation Network. He is the principal investigator for the Agency for Healthcare Research and Quality–funded Healthy Hearts in the Heartland consortium, which aims to test the capacity of primary care practices in the Midwest to improve the ABCS of cardiovascular disease prevention: aspirin in high-risk individuals, blood pressure control, cholesterol management, and smoking cessation.

Sara J. Knight, Ph.D., is a professor in preventive medicine, a division in the Department of Medicine at the University of Alabama at Birmingham, and is the director of the Health Services Research and Development Program at the Birmingham Veterans Affairs Medical Center. Her previous academic positions were at the University of California, San Francisco; Northwestern University; and The University of Chicago. From 2012 through 2014, she served as the deputy director of the national Veterans Affairs Health Services Research and Development Program.

Dr. Knight trained as a clinical health psychologist and health services researcher focusing on decision making in cancer care and genomic medicine. Her scientific expertise is in the use of mixed methods. She is an expert in the quantitative measurement of patient preferences and patient-reported outcomes, and she has a background in qualitative interview and group facilitation methods. She has experience working with large national administrative and clinical databases used to study access to care.

Throughout her career Dr. Knight has sought to understand patient and stakeholder values, goals, and preferences and patient-reported outcomes, especially in vulnerable and underserved populations. Her work has identified population-based preferences for genetic testing and has described the challenges in the organization and delivery of genomic medicine services in large health systems. Her recent work has explored ways to use community engagement to align the development of precision medicine services with the values and preferences of diverse communities.

Bruce R. Korf, M.D., Ph.D., is the Wayne H. and Sara Crews Finley Chair in Medical Genetics, a professor in and the chair of the Department of Genetics, the director of the Heflin Center for Genomic Sciences at the University of Alabama at Birmingham (UAB), and a co-director of the UAB-HudsonAlpha Center for Genomic Medicine. He is a medical geneticist, pediatrician, and child neurologist, certified by the American Board of Medical Genetics (clinical genetics, clinical cytogenetics, clinical molecular genetics), the American Board of Pediatrics, and the American Board of Psychiatry and Neurology (child neurology). Dr. Korf is the past president of the Association of Professors of Human and Medical Genetics, past president of the American College of Medical Genetics and Genomics (ACMG), and current president of the ACMG Foundation for Genetic and Genomic Medicine. He has served on the board of scientific counselors of the National Cancer Institute and the National Human Genome Research Institute at the National Institutes of Health. His major research interests are the molecular diagnosis of genetic disorders and the natural history, genetics, and treatment of neurofibromatosis. He serves as a principal investigator of the Department of Defense–funded Neurofibromatosis Clinical Trials Consortium. He is co-author of *Human Genetics and Genomics* (medical student textbook, now in its fourth edition), *Medical Genetics at a Glance* (medical student textbook, now in its third edition), *Emery and Rimoin's Principles and Practice of Medical Genetics* (now in its sixth edition), and *Current Protocols in Human Genetics*.

Debra Leonard, M.D., Ph.D., is a professor in and the chair of the Department of Pathology and Laboratory Medicine at the University of Vermont Medical Center in Burlington, Vermont. She is an expert in the molecular pathology of cancer and infectious diseases and in policy development for genomic medicine. Her M.D. and Ph.D. degrees were completed at the New York University School of Medicine, where she also did her postgraduate clinical training in anatomic pathology, including a surgical pathology fellowship. She is certified by the American Board of Pathology in Anatomic Pathology and by the American Boards of Pathology and Medical Genetics in Molecular Genetic Pathology. Currently, Dr. Leonard is a member of the National Academies of Sciences, Engineering, and Medicine's Roundtable on Genomics and Precision Health, and she previously served as a member of the Institute of Medicine's Committee on the Review of Genomics-Based Tests for Predicting Outcomes in Clinical Trials. She is a fellow of the College of American Pathologists (CAP) and the chair of the CAP's Personalized Healthcare Committee. Dr. Leonard is a past member of the Secretary's Advisory Committee on Genetics Health and Society to Secretary Michael O. Leavitt and a past president and 2009 Leadership Award recipient of the Association for Molecular Pathology. She has spoken widely on various molecular pathology test services, the future of molecular pathology, the impact of gene patents on molecular pathology, and the practice of genomic medicine.

Christine Lu, Ph.D., co-directs the Precision Medicine Translational Research (PROMoTeR) Center in the Department of Population Medicine (DPM) at Harvard Medical School. Dr. Lu leads the precision medicine and policy and the precision medicine oncology portfolios in the DPM. Her research focuses on the policy, legal, ethical, economic, and societal issues related to precision medicine, all of which have substantial impacts on the coverage and reimbursement and the clinical integration of genomic testing and sequencing. She is a multiple principal investigator of Genomics-based Technologies: Access and Reimbursement Issues. She also conducts research to assess the real-world utility of genomic testing and sequencing, including the impact of value-based contracts.

Michael Murray, M.D., is board certified in internal medicine and medical genetics, and he joined Geisinger Health System as the director of clinical genomics in 2013 after serving on the faculty at Harvard Medical School and as the clinical chief of genetics at Brigham and Women's Hospital in Boston for 9 years. Dr. Murray earned his medical degree at Penn State Hershey and went on to do additional training at the Cleveland Clinic, University of Pennsylvania, and Harvard Medical School.

At Geisinger he has led the design and implementation of the Genome-FIRST return of results program for the more than 150,000 patient participants who undergo genomic sequencing as part of the MyCode Community Health Initiative. This project builds on the collaboration between Geisinger and Regeneron Pharmaceuticals but is funded outside of that research collaboration through internal Geisinger support, external grants, and generous donations. The GenomeFIRST return of results program expects to deliver important risk information based on genetic sequence back to between 3 and 4 percent of MyCode participants in its initial phase. These risks primarily fall into the categories of either risk for cancer or cardiovascular disease. Geisinger is the first institution in the world to build the necessary infrastructure at the scale needed to deliver this kind of genomic results to this many patients and their providers and to then assist the patients in getting their at-risk family members tested too. This program is expected to help define a best practice model for doing this new 21st-century approach to care within health care systems everywhere.

Dr. Murray was one of the principal investigators on the Boston-based MedSeq project and is an investigator in both the ClinGen and eMERGE projects. He is also the lead editor of a genomics textbook for practicing clinicians, *Clinical Genomics: Practical Applications for Adult Patient Care* (McGraw-Hill, 2014).

Lori A. Orlando, M.D., M.H.S., is an associate professor of medicine, a health services researcher, and the director of the Precision Medicine Program in the Center for Applied Genomics and Precision Medicine at Duke University. She received her M.D. from Tulane University in 1998 and her M.H.S. from Duke in 2004. From 2004 to 2009 she worked with Dr. David Matchar in the Duke Center for Clinical Heath Policy Research, where she specialized in decision modeling and technology assessments. In 2009 she began working with Dr. Geoffrey Ginsburg in what is now the Center for Applied Genomics and Precision Medicine, and in 2014 she became the director of the Center's Precision Medicine Program. Her research expertise is in decision making and implementation science as they relate to identifying and managing individuals in clinical settings who are at increased risk for medical conditions. She developed MeTree, a patient-facing family health history–based risk assessment and clinical decision support program designed to facilitate the uptake of risk-stratified evidence-based guidelines in primary care. MeTree was designed to overcome the major barriers to collecting and using high-quality family health histories to guide clinical care and has been shown to be highly effective when integrated into primary care practices. In addition, her work as the director of the precision medicine program allows her to integrate expertise from across Duke to help facilitate the translation of proven precision medicine approaches, such as technologies like mHealth, SMART-FHIR, and genomics, into clinical practice.

Josh Peterson, M.D., M.P.H., is an associate professor of biomedical informatics and medicine in the School of Medicine at Vanderbilt University. Dr. Peterson's research interests are in precision medicine, with a focus on clinical decision support to improve drug safety and efficacy, and in the translation of genomic technologies to routine clinical care. He has led the design and implementation of multiple clinical decision support systems oriented toward geriatric patients, the critically ill, patients with acute and chronic kidney disease, and, most recently, for patients tested within a large pharmacogenomics implementation, PREDICT. He currently leads development and evaluation of PREDICT and serves as a principle investigator for a National Institutes of Health (NIH) Common Fund project to simulate the clinical impact and cost effectiveness of performing genomic panel testing across large populations over their lifetime. He is also active within a variety of NIH-sponsored research consortia including eMERGE, where he co-chairs the outcomes workgroup, and IGNITE, where he chairs the clinical informatics interest group. Dr. Peterson is the program director for the

Masters of Applied Clinical Informatics, which trains physicians and other health professionals in the field of clinical informatics.

Dr. Peterson received his M.D. through the Vanderbilt University School of Medicine in 1997 and completed an internal medicine residency at Duke University Medical Center, a fellowship in general internal medicine at the Brigham and Women's Hospital, and a master's of public health degree at the Harvard School of Public Health.

Bradford Powell, M.D., Ph.D., is a clinical geneticist and bioinformatician. He is an assistant professor in the Department of Genetics at the University of North Carolina (UNC) at Chapel Hill where he also directs the genetics portion of the pre-clinical curriculum for the UNC at Chapel Hill School of Medicine. As a board-certified physician in medical genetics and pediatrics, he has an active clinical practice in UNC's adult genetics and cancer genetics clinics.

Dr. Powell's research interests center on how genome-scale data are analyzed, communicated, and used in the clinical arena. He was an investigator in computational and clinical aspects with the North Carolina Clinical Genomic Evaluation by Next-generation Exome Sequencing (NCGENES) project. NCGENES studied the yield and clinical impact of diagnostic and secondary findings of genome-scale sequencing in a broad spectrum of medical conditions. He is a co-principal investigator of the successor project, NCGENES2, which will further focus on the impact of these findings in terms of clinical utility and health care use. He is also an investigator in North Carolina Newborn Exome Sequencing for Universal Screening, a project that is studying the potential impact of genetic sequencing in newborn screening.

Dean Regier, M.A., Ph.D., is a scientist at the British Columbia Cancer Agency and an assistant professor in the School of Population and Public Health at the University of British Columbia. His research focuses on cutting-edge health economics and outcomes research, particularly as they pertain to preference-based utility elicitation and health technology assessment. His current program includes the application of stated preference discrete choice experiments to health technologies and health promotion, the microeconometric analysis of discrete choice data, and probabilistic cost effectiveness and net-benefit analysis. He is particularly interested in applying preference-based techniques to estimate the personal utility and net benefit of genomic testing as it pertains to the "value of knowing," i.e., how genes may play a role in our personal lives and how patients trade among benefits, risks, and scientific uncertainties when making a treatment decision.

Richard Turner, M.A. (Cantab), M.B.B.Chir. (Cantab), MRCP(UK), is a specialist registrar in clinical pharmacology and therapeutics (CPT) with a deep interest in pharmacogenomics and precision medicine. He graduated in medicine in 2010 from the University of Cambridge. He completed his foundation training in the East of England deanery between 2010 and 2012, which included a CPT academic component investigating the pharmacogenomics of fluoropyrimidine toxicity. Dr. Turner moved to Liverpool in 2012 after being awarded a National Institute for Health Research academic clinical fellowship in CPT. During his 2 years as an academic clinical fellow he completed core medical training and was involved in a large cardiovascular pharmacogenomics study. From 2014 to 2017, Dr. Turner undertook a sustained period of doctoral research as a Medical Research Council (MRC) fellow on the North West England MRC CPT fellowship scheme, investigating the pharmacogenomics of statin-induced muscle toxicity. He has recently been awarded a Health Education England Genomics Education Programme Genomics Research and Innovation Fellowship, which will run over the next 4 years (2018–2021) alongside his continued National Health Service clinical commitments.

Appendix C

Statement of Task

An ad hoc committee will plan and conduct a 1-day public workshop to explore challenges and opportunities associated with integrating genomics into large-scale health systems or public health programs. These programs have a variety of goals, such as providing information to large segments of a given population with or without certain disease conditions about clinically actionable genetic variants, seeking diagnoses for individuals suspected to have rare diseases, and/or advancing research on the genetic contributors to human illnesses. Case studies of genomic testing programs and collaborative learning networks may be highlighted during the workshop as a way to understand successes and lessons learned regarding (1) economic considerations (e.g., clinical utility, value), (2) policy environments (e.g., alleviating privacy and discrimination concerns for participants), and (3) data sharing. Workshop discussions will be held with a broad array of stakeholders which may include health economists, representatives from health care delivery systems, public health officials, bioethicists, implementation science researchers, clinicians, payers, and policy makers. The committee will develop the workshop agenda, select and invite speakers and discussants, and may moderate the discussions. Proceedings of the workshop will be prepared by a designated rapporteur in accordance with institutional policy and procedures.

Appendix D

Registered Attendees

Joanne Adelberg
American College of Medical
    Genetics and Genomics

Megan Anderson Brooks
CRD Associates

Thalia Ashton
Pinnacle Lab Solutions

Cynthia Bens
Personalized Medicine Coalition

Gouri Shankar Bhattacharyya
Salt Lake City Medical Center,
    Kolkata

Maria Blazo
Baylor, Scott & White

Eric Boerwinkle
University of Texas Health Science
    Center; School of Public
    Health

Vence Bonham
National Human Genome Research
    Institute

Khaled Bouri
U.S. Food and Drug
    Administration

Ruth Brenner
U.S. Air Force

Tara Burke
Association for Molecular
    Pathology

Colleen Campbell
University of Iowa

Ann Cashion
National Institute of Nursing
    Research

Henry Chang
National Institutes of Health

Rex Chisholm
Northwestern University

Chetana Daniels
University of Iowa

Barry Dickinson
American Medical Association

Joe Donahue
Accenture

Emily Edelman
The Jackson Laboratory

Juvianee Estrada-Veras
Walter Reed National Military
    Medical Center

Greg Feero
*Journal of the American Medical
    Association*

Claudine Fle
AGT

Malia Fullerton
University of Washington

Arsheed Ganaie
University of Minnesota

Josh Gant
Consultant

Rachel Gatewood
University of Iowa

Gail Geller
Johns Hopkins Berman Institute of
    Bioethics

Geoff Ginsburg
Duke University

Katrina Goddard
Kaiser Permanente Center for
    Health Research

Christian Grimstein
U.S. Food and Drug
    Administration

Marc Grodman
Columbia University

Shenita-Ann Grymes
BrittNelle Health Services Group,
    LLC

Jill Hagenkord
Color Genomics

Katie Halbmaier
University of Iowa College of
    Nursing

Jeffrey Hankoff
Cigna

Ragan Hart
University of Washington

Lydia Hellwig
Uniformed Services University of
    the Health Sciences

Jonathan Holt
Physician

Gillian Hooker
Concert Genetics

Carol Horowitz
Icahn School of Medicine at
    Mount Sinai

Geoffrey Hymans
Department of Health and Human
  Services

George Isham
HealthPartners

Nicole Johnson
Hayes, Inc.

Darlene Kaskie
National Network of Libraries of
  Medicine

Amy Kennedy
National Cancer Institute

Abel Kho
Northwestern University

Muin Khoury
Centers for Disease Control and
  Prevention

Shannon Kirkland
National Education Association

Elizabeth Kiscaden
National Network of Libraries of
  Medicine, Greater Midwest
  Region

Sara Knight
University of Alabama at
  Birmingham

Bruce Korf
University of Alabama at
  Birmingham

Alyson Krokosky
Walter Reed National Military
  Medical Center

Jennifer Krupp
American College of Medical
  Genetics and Genomics

Katherine Lambertson
Genetic Alliance

Erin Lambie
The George Washington University

Kristofor Langlais
National Institutes of Health

Gabriela Lavezzari
Biocerna

Grace Lawrence
Inova Genomics Laboratory

David Ledbetter
Geisinger Health System

Debra Leonard
University of Vermont Medical
  Center

Elissa Levin
Helix

Srisuporn Lidla
Six Senses Yao Noi

David Litwack
U.S. Food and Drug
  Administration

Christine Lu
Harvard Medical School

Teri Manolio
National Human Genome
  Research Institute

Monique Mansoura
Massachusetts Institute of
  Technology

Jennifer McCormick
The Pennsylvania State University

Victoria Menzies
Virginia Commonwealth University

Rana Morris
National Center for Biotechnology
  Information

Michael Murray
Geisinger Health System

Hiromi Ono
National Institutes of Health

Lori Orlando
Duke University

Michael Pacanowski
U.S. Food and Drug
  Administration

Peggy Peissig
Marshfield Clinic Research
  Institute

Michelle Penny
Biogen

Josh Peterson
Vanderbilt University Medical
  Center

Bradford Powell
University of North Carolina at
  Chapel Hill

Vicky Pratt
Association for Molecular
  Pathology

Daryl Pritchard
Personalized Medicine Coalition

Natalie Pritchett
National Cancer Institute

Ronald Przygodzki
Department of Veterans Affairs

Erica Ramos
National Society of Genetic
  Counselors

Dean Regier
B.C. Cancer Agency/University of
  British Columbia

Karina Reyes Gordillo
The George Washington University

Megan Roberts
National Cancer Institute

Carol Robertson-Plouch
Biopharmaceutical Advisors and
  Consultants

Laura Lyman Rodriguez
National Human Genome
  Research Institute

Sarah Savage
FDNA

Brock Schroeder
Illumina, Inc.

Sheri Schully
National Institutes of Health

Joan Scott
Health Resources and Services
　Administration

Geetha Senthil
National Institute of Mental
　Health

Sam Shekar
Northrop Grumman Information
　Systems

Nonniekaye Shelburne
National Cancer Institute

Lily Silayeva
The Tauri Group

Sikha Singh
Association of Public Health
　Laboratories

Angela Starkweather
University of Connecticut

Casey Overby Taylor
Johns Hopkins University

Zivana Tezak
U.S. Food and Drug
　Administration

Wendy Toler
Consultant

Scott Topper
Color Genomics

Clesson Turner
Walter Reed National Military
　Medical Center

Richard Turner
University of Liverpool

Dila Udum
Bahcesehir University

Dave Veenstra
University of Washington

Rashi Venkataraman
America's Health Insurance Plans

Linda Walton
University of Iowa

Catharine Wang
Boston University

Michael Watson
American College of Medical
　Genetics and Genomics

Meredith Weaver
American College of Medical
　Genetics and Genomics

Catherine Wicklund
National Society of Genetic
　Counselors

David Wierz
The OCI Group

Janet Williams
American Academy of Nursing/
　University of Iowa

Jennifer Wilson
Stanford University

Theresa Wizemann
Wizemann Scientific
　Communications, LLC

Kenn Wong
Counsyl

Grant Wood
Intermountain Healthcare

Guisou Zarbalian
Association of Public Health
    Laboratories